The Silence of the Body

TRANSLATED FROM THE ITALIAN BY

MICHAEL MOORE

Farrar, Straus and Giroux

New York

THE SILENCE

OF THE BODY

Materials for the Study

of Medicine

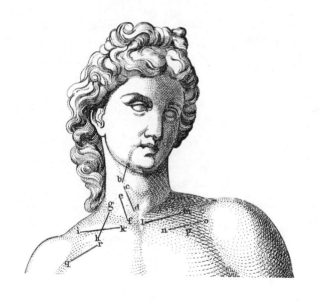

GUIDO

CERONETTI

Translation © *1993* by Michael Moore
Originally published in Italian as Il Silenzio del corpo:
Materiali per studio di medicina (fifth edition, May *1990*), ©
1979 Adelphi edizioni s.p.a. Milano
All rights reserved
Printed in the United States of America
Published simultaneously in Canada by HarperCollinsCanadaLtd
Designed by Cynthia Krupat
First edition, *1993*

Library of Congress Cataloging-in-Publication Data
Ceronetti, Guido.
[Silenzio del corpo. English]
The silence of the body: materials for the study of medicine /
Guido Ceronetti; translated from the Italian by Michael Moore. —
1st ed.
p. cm.
1. Medicine—Philosophy. 2. Body, Human. I. Title.
R723.C43613 *1993*   610'.1—dc20   93-21641   CIP

Glorify God in your body.

—I CORINTHIANS 6:20

The Silence of the Body

My entire study of medicine is contained in this collection of yellowed clippings—excerpts, abstracts, and glosses of other people's ideas—and tainted memories of dreams, of human contact. It pokes its way through a crack in the wall between two different figures. On one side sits the umbilical, radiant Buddha, King of Physicians, as he is called, whom I could never have been; on the other hangs an old print of an authoritative, learned, and beloved provincial doctor (though one not nearly as busy as Bénassis, Balzac's boring philanthropist), whom I would like to have been, with a nice house and small garden in a Europe sometime between the discovery of the smallpox vaccine and the first aspirin. Or it slips down a drainpipe between the good family caretaker who has disappeared from our bedsides, where childbirth, sickness, and death now find it indecent to visit us, and the Gnostic thaumaturge, the mesmeric toucher, the Yajur-Vedic healer, the Hippocratic diagnostician, the anthroposophic soother, the homeopathic restabilizer, the Chinese needle thrower, the macrobiotic dietitian.

Traditionally, Medicine is a philosophical discipline that can be studied in any number of ways, going to medical school among

*them. But no one can stop us from opening up the human skull,
heart, or stomach in solitude, from reading the threads that tie
man to the heavens and to the chthonic regions, and from curing
ourselves or allowing ourselves to die, to be cured of life, alone.
I am a physician in my search for the truth, and the truth is
always therapeutic, masterfully surgical, and splendidly philanthropic. My limits are the same as those of any ordinary medical
practitioner who gropes through the debilitating appearances of
life and death and the infinite disguises of our overlapping
realities—these pensive, erratic creations of the body's catalogues
of sensations.*

These fragments are the disjecta membra *of an elusive, cov-
eted, and vaguely scented knowledge. I have extracted them from
the darkness of entombed notebooks, where they had been buried
for future use and pleasure under the inscription "Medicine."
Sometimes they were the catalysts for a curious man's erudite
adventures and disinterested probings. For I am as happy to rum-
mage through the human microcosm (and proclaim in the face of
stupidity and silence that it is* divine *and* tragic) *as I am to grasp
or define nothing with rigorous certainty, except its divine and
tragic essence. Once you have grasped the silence of the body,
dissecting or overstepping its limits by some interior light, the trip
back is a gloomy one. The extraordinary voyages made into this
silence by Lucretius, Leonardo, and Bichat all ended against the
inanimate cliffs of an Atlantis submerged for infinity.*

*The body? Here are its ashes, scattered to the wind by an
uninterrupted pursuit of knowledge. The agonizing, innocent dual-
ism of body and soul is resuscitated by every sublime harmonious
sound, by every voice of supreme calm, and by every echo of the
god's movements in this mute theater. The eyes that flee from the
decomposed figure (it's in the next room, it's at the bottom of the
stairs, it's on the sidewalk) can repress the sight by shifting back
and forth between an appearance that is not all and an all that is
only apparent as we wait for the skies to open and reveal what
this symbol, this body symbol, symbol of symbols, was saying.*

The Silence of the Body

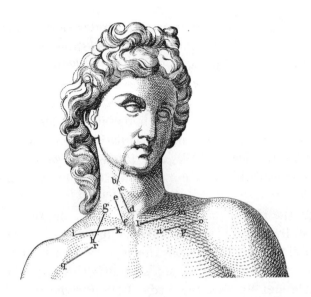

My brother, my sister. This is what ancient lovers would call each other, not to disguise their snare or to make it more tender, more morbid, but in imitation of the divine couples, of the distant endogamy from which we all descend. But where esogamy was the rule, the same expressions could sound quite erotic in a prohibited relationship. As Martial says: You call your mother sister, so for you she is neither mother nor sister.

Male lovers were *fratres*, a specialty of monasteries and fraternities (*Si triduo sine fratre dormieris*—if you sleep without your "brother" for three days [Petronius, 129]). Female lovers were *sorores*—the meeting of two sharp edges, of four feverish and evil eyes. This was not always so: there was a time of fat pigeons and trout. "Et sa soeur, les mains sur ses seins, la baise"—And her sister, hands on her breasts, kisses her (Verlaine).

In Apollinaire's "C'est un petit soldat mon frère et mon amant," *frère* is ambiguous because the trenches and home are linked (especially in wartime) by pure brotherhood. Among the great tragedies of childhood, De Quincey included that of the little boy's lips forever separated from his sister's kisses. Men with no sisters also share in this tragedy. Gloomy, incessant *death of the sister* in Munch's paintings. (Without a dead sister, abandoned lifeless at the foot of a distant staircase, a man cannot rediscover in the dark his sister's lips, the good wound happy to start bleeding again.) At its most ethereal and imaginative, a sister's wedding reaches the deepest endogamic intensity; it makes us feel as if our ties with Chaos and the contracted universe cannot be undone.

In the Hindu *Rig-Veda* (X, 14), Yami, the sister, unsuccessfully tempts her brother, Yama, to become her *frater* ("Let us roll together like wagon wheels"). He replies that it is not right to uncover one's sister's nudity; this is prohibited by Mitra and Varuna, the Vedic Elohim, who spy on men's actions. Yami is enraged by his rejection, but less than Phaedra. (Yami is an example of chastity, by contrast with Phaedra's *incestos amores*.)

In all pornographic literature, high and low, Yami renews her attack and triumphs easily; she is Tiamat victorious over Marduk, Chaos digging its claws into order, the cosmos, the Torah, Manu. Brother, my brother, whisper the tenebrous Great Waters. Yami's victories, over even the most punitive mores, are frequent and probably more numerous than her defeats. No one can count them . . . They are hidden by the night and by walls that spies cannot penetrate. With the end of myth, Mitra and Varuna may have become indifferent to seemingly ordinary cases. But to maintain order, a condemnation of Yami's excesses will suffice; her armor cannot be breached until it is noisily removed. What a fool calls *hypocrisy* simply provides nurture for the balance of the human world, the only known respite in our race toward disintegration.

•

The Silence of the Body

In some cities of the world, anything goes. They are like public baths or brothels established by the gods, where you go to be free from all limits. Alexandria was one such place: *Athenis dimidium licet, Alexandriae totum*—In Athens you can go halfway, in Alexandria all the way (Seneca, *Apocolocyn-thosis*). So it must have been in the late nineteenth century, but Cavafy morbidly pretended that he was surrounded and tormented by a puritanical society. He left the lamps in his house unlit, the better to toy with his memories and *forbidden images*.

In the West, Paris was the *énorme catin*, the great whore (Baudelaire). Rimbaud inherited Baudelaire's vision of the 1871 Communard revolt as a heroic (and thoroughly mis-guided) attempt to be purified of, and released from, the city's ferment (socialist revolts annul the license granted by the gods). But there is something sad about cities where Eros turns into an evil tyrant. (Sodom is a mythic example of how asphyxiating extreme freedom can be: fire rained down to free it.) Paris was ruled by Nana, the epitome of absolute por-nocracy: "Invisible, floating above the ball on her supple limbs, she decomposed this world, piercing it with the fer-ment of her scent wafting on the hot air, to the vulgar rhythm of the music." Poetry is the angels' reward to places chosen for boundless fermentation—like a formal constraint, a ritual enchantment, a Latin *carmen*, a paradoxical freedom from the tyranny of excessive pleasure that torments their inhabitants.

·

The Vulgar Latin word for liver is *ficatum*, because geese, with their fat livers, were fed a diet of figs (*ficus*). Thus a noble organ (perhaps the noblest of them all: the brain's nobility is questionable) took its name from mankind's ancient iniquity. There is a smattering of blood at the origins of everything human.

"They're as quiet as an ass getting shaved," said Burchiello, a barber. I think he meant that, out of respect for the person shaving it, the ass tries not to bray.

.

Shortly before his death, Shelley often saw a man whose huge black cloak turned him into a silhouette; with irresistible power, the man would entice him to follow. All at once the cloak would fall and Shelley would see himself in the other man, who sneered and said, "Now are you satisfied?"

.

A medieval sentence defends the rights of the penis: *Quod turget, urget*—What swells, impels. It sternly equates these rights with those of the abscess and the pimple.

.

I found the idea for my story "The Women of Pompeii" in Buret's *Le Gros mal du Moyen Âge et la syphilis actuelle* (1894). He claims that sex with priapi was one of the most common causes for the spread of venereal disease. Maybe this explains Martial's two mysterious verses on the woods of Anna Perenna.* The butt ends of broomsticks in the trammeled female Eros, toothpaste tubes in a pornographic magazine. Contagion, however, was the work of a god.

.

I am thin, very thin, extremely thin, and I can become even thinner, and thinner still, until I fly out the window. But

---

* "*Et quod virgineo cruore gaudet / Annae pomiferum nemus Perennae.*" The tree-bearing grove of Anna Perenna / that takes delight in virgin gore. IV, 64.

the thought of this spiritual metamorphosis into an angelic butterfly makes me nostalgic for the chrysalis. I want my earthly weight back, so I echo Scarron's cry:

Revenez mes fesses perdues
Revenez me donner un cul.

(Bring me back the butt I lack
Bring me back my purloined ass.)

•

The Italians thought that the Longobards, the *rea progenie*, all had bad breath. "Don't marry Hermengard," Pope Stephen III wrote to Charlemagne, "she stinks like all the Longobards." Charlemagne married her anyway and ended up repudiating her; he couldn't stand her stench. Manzoni conceals the truth in his play *Adelchi*, although he was certainly aware of it. The sixth book of Andrea da Barberino's *I Reali di Francia* talks about the wedding of King Pepin to Bertha the Longobard (Big-foot Bertha—better an oversized right foot than a bad odor), but it does not allude to this inconvenience. Instead, Bertha was disgusted by King Pepin: "She remembered her mother had told her that he was old but not how uncouth he was in his person or how foul; and all the while one could see her sorrow by the way her face changed."

The Roman Emperor Marcus Aurelius bragged that his Hungarian legionnaires stank less than the Jews, but when the Longobards moved from Buda to Pavia, their breath may have turned foul.

•

When Jacques de Cambry visited Quimperlé in lower Brittany during the Reign of Terror, he learned that the *Caqueux* had been outlawed and were now treated as untouchables (*Voyage dans le Finistère*). They had been sorcerers and soothsayers, and on Holy Friday blood issued from their navels. But after the French Revolution, their navels dried up.

.

You eat in company but fast in solitude, because the breath of someone who is fasting turns foul. *Numquid spiritus ieiunio marcet?*—Do I have bad breath because of not having eaten? (Petronius, 128).

.

One tradition says the Antichrist will be born by cesarean section. Countless babies are born this way today. One of them is the Antichrist, but it is hard to tell which. In the future it could be *almost* anyone; we shall know the Antichrist has arrived, and his name is *Everyone*.

.

A woman suffering from lupus, with a disfigured face, suddenly runs into a group of people who are talking about her. Upon seeing her, all of them are struck dumb. *Lupus in fabula*—Speak of the devil.

.

The long life of the mummy through human plagues and purulences. *Mum* is a Persian pharmacological term, meaning wax or balm. *Mumiyah* is Arabic for asphalt. Arab desecraters dug up these masses of asphalt and petrified but still active resins and sold them as a panacea (for ulcers, war wounds, fractures, anemia, hemoptysis, incontinence, migraines, paralysis, nervous tics, epilepsy, coughs, and otitis). Business was good, because the product was expensive. But they quickly ran out of real mummies, so traffic in fake mummies began, with little respect for the dead and their grief. Arab

Egypt began to fabricate mummies from corpses snatched off the streets or robbed from graveyards at the risk of beatings.

Ambroise Paré relates that the King of Navarre's physician, Guy de la Fontaine, visited a Palestinian's warehouse in Alexandria, where forty mummies in gelatin had just been fabricated. He mentions that they were also being made in the West, from bodies cut down from the gallows, dried in an oven, and dipped in tar. Mummies were sold in little jars each containing a small piece of human flesh candied in asphalt and in antiseptic resins (very similar to our own canned meat). Though lacking the antiquity and prestige of the hypogeum, the fake mummy was ultimately more of a mummy than the ones that had been asleep for thousands of years.

Once the end had come to this collective illusion—a drug's most active ingredient—the drug was no longer a therapeutic mummy and ended up in the museum of pharmacy. Today we have the chemotherapy mummy, the antibiotic mummy, the cortisone mummy, the radioactive mummy, and countless other mummies in jars. The basic ingredient is always a little bit of human flesh, in a variety of forms. (With profound psychology, homeopathy reduces the active ingredient to almost nothing, buffering both the drug's efficiency and its danger and weakening it through dilution after dilution.) And note the importance of asphalt, yesterday's great mummy and medicine of the body and, for a century now, the great mummy and medicine of the economy. Asphalt supplies *energy*—no small thing—but in its overwhelming growth, nourished till it becomes human flesh and blood, it reveals its true face as mineral dominator of the world, destroyer of life.

•

"Bread is bad, eat little of it," recommended Céline at a time when ordinary bread was still good. Bread is ambiguous, like everything it compares to and symbolizes. It contains yeast, and without yeast it would not be bread. But yeast is a cadaveric impurity, a living death. The flight from Egypt with the Passover matzo symbolizes the desire to leave behind every trace of death. We can reread Exodus in light of the matzo . . . The Jewish family as a fleeing matzo that cannot be captured by the Angel of Death's transforming yeast . . . Moses and Aaron knew the secrets of the living and of the dead. Yeast is the Angel of Death, and matzo is a dove seeking shelter from death across the Sea of Reeds, far from the black land where the Egyptians, the children of Khem, delve into death and make bread, for the living and the dead, in their ovens of fiery darkness.

The tenth plague, death of the firstborn sons, *pesach* is what Exodus calls the silence of the yeast surrounding the flight of the Jewish matzo. Either a story of doors bolted by an epidemic or a symbolic silence that hides the mystery of yeast, of the abhorred death, in the work of the baker and the brewer, who come and go from house to tomb. No army chases after the poor ragged souls who follow these two violent sacerdotal princes, as no dogs howled that night in Egypt, so as not to disturb the perfect silence in which destinies were separated and a doctrine was sacrilegiously amputated.

The army is imaginary. The only real thing is death, nesting in the leavened bread, *chametz*, a word that contains the idea of violence. The matzo people flee the yeast army, celebrating an illusory triumph over the need for death. Passover is the destruction, by candlelight, of all yeast in the house: Babylonian polenta, Median beer, Idumaean vinegar, Egyptian beer, dyers' compounds, bakers' dough, scribes' glue (*Pesachim*). The enemy of Passover is yeast, the dark, powerful element suggested to Egyptian bakers by their continuous handling of corpses. It will reappear, carrying the contagion

The Silence of the Body

of death, in the leavened bread Jesus Christ, resurrected by yeast to say the Exodus was useless and "The Pharaoh's army is here." The Jewish mistake and miracle is the refusal to mix with death; this prevents the Jews from experiencing a true spiritual transcendence and instead roots them in human time *dor-va-dor*, until the end of the world.

An oven for Egyptian bread, shaped like a truncated cone, was the first alchemist's oven; its hermetic *nigredo*, teeming with live bacteria, was the yeast. Bread was born in Egypt, where the meeting of food and death, of a dead man and his need for nourishment, resembles the meeting of dough and yeast. The dead man is the yeast of an unknown bread, rising in the boat-ovens of his exodus into infinity and into the clots and crusts, the future medicine, of his mummy.

Thus Céline, a metaphysical *practicien*, was right. Bread is *bad* for you (the better, the truer bread is, the worse it is for you), and a diet based on corn, spelt, oats, rice, and matzo is better: it contains more life. Bread should be eaten only once a year, and matzo every day. But to stretch Passover out too much, for hygienic reasons, would defile what has been handed down to us as Scripture. It would annul the mysterious sign, which has yet to be understood. In reality we are condemned to eat bread, we heirs of Egypt, children and slaves of the oven. It is right for our main food to be a product of human effort containing both light and darkness, symbolizing life raised from death, eaten today only by the living, but a product that for a thousand years many times over has been on the table of the dead.

·

Hippocrates learned medicine from Egypt, a shelter housing all the infectious diseases. Imhotep's bag never had a moment's rest. Out of it came beautiful surgical instruments and an anesthetic made from vinegar and the dust of Memphis marble, to treat every type of tumor listed in the Ebers papyrus. Perhaps the same diseases existed in Rome and Athens, but Egypt in particular conjures up the image of a sad, sick man and of a wisdom in the shadow of his disease, smelling of iodine and camphor, at the end of a gray ward in an old hospital. (The Romans had instead a cheerful sanatorium whose dry climate attracted everyone who coughed.) Blame it on the museums; they exhibit only ruins from tombs, and welcome you with a long moan, interrupted by the barking of Anubis.

Like intelligent people who suffer from chronic illnesses, the Egyptians were mischievous, humorous, and satiric. The Nile was their perpetual and colossal physician, with the gods in charge of the various wards, followed by throngs of assistants. Professor Bes and his wife, Tueris, supervised births to ensure that newborns were correctly deformed: he was a dropsical dwarf, hairy and bearded; she a behemoth fresh from the woods.

So much rachitis! So many backs with Pott's disease! So many spastics! So many dystrophics! So many blind and half-blind! Polio, smallpox, typhus, leprosy, bilharziasis, cholera . . . They got drunk for relief, and their bellies swelled with liquid . . . I imagine Egypt as a giant freak show of curved spinal columns, achondroplastics, irregular outlines, and exsanguine profiles, under the protection of dogs, cats, crocodiles, hippopotami, oxen, and monstrous chimeras, the only ones to possess good health in the Nile Valley. And the parasites, permanent guests of the bowels: *pend, heft, herxetf,* the ruthless corroding worms, the tapeworm, the duodenal Ancylostoma, the Schistosoma haematobium (less prevalent than today, however, because there were throngs of ibis which devoured the bilharzia eggs in shellfish), and the worm of *àààà,* the unknown disease . . . Endless torrents of diarrhea . . .

The Silence of the Body

Various authors deny there was syphilis: hard to believe, although the mummies, when asked, replied in the negative. But in the Hellenistic age, syphilis was too widespread to have spared Ptolemaic Egypt. (Giovanni Marro studied a suspect gumma caries in a Ptolemaic skull at the Egyptian museum in Turin.)

I am amazed that such big onion eaters were so diced by infectious diseases . . . Famously flatulent . . . But at least their kidneys worked . . . Bread and beer swelled the stomachs—the *rohet*—of the poor, the bellies of the peasants; game meat and roast gazelle or ostrich inflamed the stomachs of the rich. A people deeply immersed in the mystery of nourishment: they received it from a river god, shared it with the dead and with the heavenly beings, with the breath of the living universe. They mated Kitchen and Tomb to invent bread and alchemy. If an invoked deity refused to heal a sick person, the supreme threat of the man of words was: You won't get any more to eat.

•

Famous mistakes of Greek medicine, later adopted and disseminated by Arab physicians: the bifurcated uterus, the existence of growths to nourish the uterine mucous membrane, the migration of the uterus inside the body (Meyerhof, *La Gynécologie et l'obstétrique chez Avicenne et leurs rapports avec celles des Grecs*, 1938). Both the imaginative Plato and Hippocrates believed in the migration of the uterus, an animal eager to mate, whose craving for semen made it travel from one part of the body to the other, provoking Hysteria; but this is only a way of saying that, like every other living creature, the female body travels inside the uterus.

•

Albert Camus said to Jean Guitton, "He never killed a fly." Guitton replied, "The fly he didn't kill carried the plague elsewhere." He should have said flea rather than fly, but the moral is the same.

.

Jews and neurosis. In the *Leçons du mardi à la Salpetrière*, Charcot said: "Among the Jews, as I have told you again and again, nervous pathology is often, and more than elsewhere, richly represented; in particular, under excellent study conditions, one can observe in their great families the varied associations that can form the arthritic element and the nervous element." (Charcot had also studied nervous phenomena among the Sephardic Jews of the mellah in Tétouan, Morocco, where he found the same combinations of hereditary neurosis and arthritis.)

.

In the sixth book of *De Medicina*, Celsus advised rest and hot sitz baths for hemorrhoids. Then, while sitting in the hot bath, one peels two hard-boiled eggs (from a pigeon) and gently begins to stroke the ailing part first with one egg, then with the other. Gentleness for our poor ass! *Anus quoque multa taediique plena mala recipit*—The anus is host to many ills that are quite disgusting . . .

.

Non venit ad duros pallida Cura toros—Pale Care comes not to hard beds (Martial, XIV, 162). She does come there, though. Perhaps to keep her from coming, the beds need to be even harder. They should be beds of nails, on top of which we lie naked. Care will open the door halfway, see us bleeding, and turn back.

.

The Silence of the Body

The glans was red as liver, and when it swelled it took the shape of an inverted heart—monstrous—whose tip oozed drops of blood.

.

Nice title: *The convulsions of ladies of* bel esprit, *of ladies with a fondness for literature, and of others afflicted by the sweet passion of love, a disease of this century. With the anatomy of some of their hearts and brains,* by Giovanni Virani, 1789. What an appropriate year to study convulsions!

.

Interesting observation in a study of Judaism and alcoholism: Alcoholism is rare in Jewish communities in the United States (*Revue d'Histoire de la Médicine Hébraïque*, March 1957). Alcoholic intoxication increases, however, at the same rate as orthodoxy decreases. For the modern Jew, alcohol may be a Dionysian surrogate for Abraham's abstemious God. In dying from alcoholism, Joseph Roth pointed to that other God.

.

Dried dates, says Maimonides, give you migraines. But the pleasure of a date gives joy to the heart.

.

American gynecologists, says Professor Baruk, have found that cancer of the cervix and of the penis are extremely rare among observant Jews, because they completely abstain from coitus during menstruation and because circumcision eliminates smegma and its carcinogenic effects. Even at the 1963 Moscow conference on cancer, cervical carcinoma was said to be quite rare among circumcised populations, a sign that the baptized do not bother washing off smegma. Littré defined smegma as a "whitish substance, with the consistency of wet soap, which accumulates in the folds of the genital organs."

17

One might poetically call it "the soap that does not cleanse." Uterine blood is highly symbolic: life-death . . . Like a sacred event it burns the fingers. To proclaim it innocuous on the basis of material analyses was imprudent, a reckless gamble . . .

•

In *Voyage chez les lépreux*, Zambaco Pacha tells this story: "A very pretty girl from a good family fell madly in love with a man in the initial stages of leprosy and was able to marry him, since marriage with a leper or between lepers was not forbidden in Samos. This woman lived with her husband for eight years. Out of jealousy and selfishness, he strove to transmit the disease to her by every means possible; he did not want her to survive him. He was forever kissing her on the mouth, slipping her his tongue to kiss for hours, since he already had huge ulcers on his palate . . . He infected her with leprosy over and over again. All to no avail. The woman is still alive, safe and sound."

Eight years of leperous caresses (lepers are very lecherous) with one goal only—to die together in a single living decomposition—and yet failure, defeat by a microorganism's refusal to contaminate. Looking at herself in the mirror to detect the signs, she discovers to her horror that her skin is still intact! She overcame every disgust in order to be infected, and behold, her sacrifice was useless: her leper wastes away by himself. To be fair, she did not kill herself, because she wanted to die from his same illness. She loved leprosy more than the leper.

•

Either skeptics or septics.

•

The Silence of the Body

Incendium mundi. Destruction of the biosphere's protective strata, raw sunlight, *solvet saeclum in favilla.* Alone in chasms of darkness, a solitary cell masturbates, like Atum-Ra, and begets another. Multiplication. In a billion years, more or less, life becomes possible again at some point. The cell forms complete organisms. Two animals couple under Yucatán rains. Mushrooms as high as mountains. Monstrous carnivorous trees. Huge proboscises emerge from the water. A billion years more and behold Sophocles, Alexander, Lucretius, Caesar, the famous lovers, the great murderers, Copernicus, Sade, Freud, Einstein, Nuclear Energy, the end. *Leti sub dentibus ipsis*—in the very teeth of death. Throughout this constant swallowing and spewing of worlds without reality, man dreams about the *rationality* and *wisdom* of history.

•

The whole world, claimed Forbes-Winslow, Victorian alienist and criminologist, is irremediably destined to become mad unless we radically change our current style of life.

•

Optimism is like carbon monoxide; it leaves a rosy imprint on the cadaver when it kills.

•

As long as they have the wish to kill, they will not lose the lust to procreate.

•

"C'est l'heure où les douleurs des malades s'aigrissent"— Now is the time the pains of the sick grow sharper (Baudelaire, *Crépuscle du soir*). Baudelaire suffered these pains, since osteitic discomfort and syphilitic headaches increase at night. De La Martinière describes the earth's malignant vapors, which are drawn to the human body and stir its humors: "La raison pourquoi l'humeur vérolique s'esmeut le soir et cesse le jour—The reason the luetic humor stirs in the evening and abates in the day" (*Traité de la maladie vénérienne*, 1664). Baudelaire depicts his pain in *Voyage à Cythère*: "J'ai senti tous les becs et toutes les mâchoires—I felt every beak and every jaw." Evening as the opposite of what Foscolo calls *fatal quïete*: an image not of death but of exasperation with *mal de vivre*, living body of Angra Mainyu.

Not even demigods like Alcides can escape the earth's malignant vapors. "Les poisons de la terre infectent le sang reçu des immortels—The earth's poisons infect the blood received from the immortals," says Maurice de Guérin's *Centaure*. The shirt of Nessus was dipped in luetic humor and delivered by a woman. I suspect it represents the caul through whose sleeve we all are born (except cesareans). Heracles saves himself from the poison's burning by throwing himself into the pyre.

In Toltec myth, the god Centeotl Inopiltzin (Orphan God, Alone, Fatherless) invites the wise man Nanahuatzin (called *el Sabio* and *el Buboso*), who has long suffered the pains that grow sharper at night, to throw himself into the fire. El Buboso throws himself, a beautiful eagle descended from heaven carries him up, and the syphilitic wise man turns into the Sun (infected star, spotted star—the spots are Nanahuatzin's boils—and the sun writhes with pain when it sets).

Thus the light that nourishes the living blends wisdom and horror and carries the pains and metamorphoses of twilight ("Et l'homme impatient se change en bête fauve—And the impatient man becomes a beast of prey"). Giuseppe Parini's poem "Night" opens with a perfect intuition of nocturnal reality, not as deprivation of light but as the *subjugation* of the remaining natural (and artificial) light. Through infinite struggles, human civilization succeeds in dominating the Buboes, using medicines and hygiene to defeat the disease of Deinara's tunic and of the righteous man from Uz. But who will cure the syphilis in the blood of the Sun? Who can stop the night, which comes back to infect us every twelve hours?

.

Maybe Gilles de Rais should have been put in an asylum and asked to make collages at the first sign of the craving for orgies and massacres seething within him. He would have found an outlet for his madness and been cured. His extraordinary collages would have sparked endless discussions. He would have been reborn as an artist who carried the seed of great crimes. But we would never have known that he carried them, just as we do not know how much crime is contained and submerged in the expiating *ergon* of certain great artists who never cease to amaze.

.

Pascal observed that Plato and Aristotle wrote about politics only to lay down the law in a madhouse.

.

Socrates advised young people to look at themselves in the mirror often, for when they saw their beauty they would make themselves worthy of it (*axioi gignointo*). In my notebook, below this Socratic maxim, I find a strange comment from Fargue, fallen there by chance: "Sa voix sort de son suspensoir—His voice rises from his jockstrap."

.

A woman has a very big dog that loves her and is extremely jealous. She brings little kittens into the house and covers them with caresses. After a brief and difficult cohabitation, the dog slaughters them. Thus she has proof of his love: she has made a murderer out of him.

·

In the world of love, repulsion is more frequent and important than attraction. Like two sheets of paper held together by a strong glue, drifting on an ocean of boiling water.

·

Émile Mauchamp (murdered in Marrakech, 1907) says that in the Judaism of Maghreb, the devil has a much greater role than the Divinity. In the mellah the sorcerer has more prestige and credibility than a rabbi (*La Sorcellerie au Maroc*).

·

Mauchamp: If an expectant mother sees a naked woman who makes her wish for a girl, or a naked man who makes her wish for a boy, and in that moment, pregnant with a child of the opposite sex, she scratches her vulva, a hermaphrodite will be born. To prevent such a mishap, do not speak of the snake's deadly bite (speak rather of its living, vital bite: *el kerset el haya*).

On the eve of the Sabbath, one mustn't say words like egg, needle, coal, and scissors, but in their place one should say the hen's child, the key, the apple, the exact. Palm readers examine a man's right hand and a woman's left, otherwise the reading is false. A child who laughs in its sleep is dreaming that its father is dying. To get rid of nightmares: For three consecutive mornings, put your hand in the toilet after pouring a little oil in it; then place your hand over your stomach. Remain in this position all day, drinking water the blacksmith used to cool a red-hot poker.

When two women make love there is no oral contact, only generous rubbing of vulvas (Brantôme's *fricarelle*). Billy-goat testicle, called the Companion of Solitude, is in such high demand for female masturbation that butchers are forbidden to sell it whole: they have to split it in two to make it innocent. Ladies-in-waiting are allowed to have only carrots and beets that have been sliced. To make a woman sterile dip the sharp edge of a knife in her menstrual discharge and bury the knife in a cemetery: she will be sterile as long as it stays buried. She will become permanently sterile if she eats grains of barley fallen from the mouth of a she-mule and soaked in her menstrual blood. A small piece of alum in the vagina turns sperm into water, but a newly circumcised baby's foreskin, eaten raw, causes pregnancy. To inflict a woman with uncontrollable discharges, get her to swallow the powder of seven leeches dried in a tube. The remedy is a laxative of rancid melted butter.

A mutilated crow, wrapped in bay leaves and black cloth and buried in an ancient tomb, causes perpetual paralysis. The earth is a minefield of bundles containing hexes that strike the intended victims as they walk over them. (This terrifying earth sprouts fears of going out, of walking, and the Psalms' pleas for deliverance.) But the remedy for bad dreams—to immediately tell them to the toilet—is highly rational. Telling your dream to the toilet purges you; it unburdens the mind as you unburden the body, and in the proper place. I have been practicing this method for years and recommend it to anyone who is not superstitious. This practice should be applied to all kinds of mental constipation: libidos, fanaticisms, loves, bereavements, painful memories, fears, manias, ambitions, etc. Lock yourself in the bathroom and purge yourself. Confess to the great ear-hole, which will not reveal anything to anyone. The toilet is an honest doctor and a faithful friend.

·

This is what is so immoral about the much lauded *conscious* procreation. The crime of *making a man*, of bringing more evil and sorrow into the world, is not committed unconsciously in dramatic ecstasy, in the darkness of copulation; it is coldly premeditated. The usual precautions are temporarily banished, and repeated attempts are made until the goal has been achieved. Even worse is artificial procreation, with its frozen semen. To prevent the manipulator and the subject womb from being horrified by what they are doing, they abolish the *heat of the moment*, the *voluptas* that would make it a little easier.

.

I was floating blissfully on a river of shit, my arms opened wide, until I ejaculated. (The river of shit that gives pleasure is Life; although it may assume the appearance of pure water, it is still Maya in one of her disguises.)

.

It's not what you eat but what you don't eat that is good for both the body and the soul.

.

From *La Médecine en désarroi* (1938), by the once famous Dr. Kopaczewsky. He says that in the First World War German doctors used normal horse serum against diphtheria (because it was impossible to manufacture the huge quantities of vaccine needed) with the same recovery rate they would have obtained with a specific anti-diphtheria serum. In the Russo-Japanese War, the Japanese preferred bandages soaked in Peruvian balsam (a weak antiseptic, according to pharmacologists) over anti-tetanus serum. Since Kopaczewsky distrusted vaccines, he did not like transfusions (he wrote a work arguing against transfusions, *Transfusion de sang*, 1925).

He is a charming skeptic: "Deafening publicity is currently trumpeting the effectiveness of onion juice against cancer, simply because the disease is rare among Jews, who are great onion eaters." Alimentary Marranism must have considerably lowered Jewish consumption of onions. Cancer, which was unknown to old Palestine, swarms like Samson's bees in today's Israel. In any case, onions everywhere are radiating cobalt 60! Buy nonradiated onions and eat plenty of them: they guard against everything except certain hexes. Kidney problems, asthma, diarrhea, constipation, hepatitis, pimples . . . I have an onionologist's prescription for treating nervous fits: Cut an onion in two and inhale deeply. Other texts expressly prescribe garlic as a prophylactic against cancer. Clearly those who eat neither garlic nor onions deprive themselves of two formidable shields.

Kopaczewsky on the unpredictability of bacteriological reactions: "All reactions based on the hypothetical specificity of microbes and on the strange immutability of their characteristics are worthless, to be discarded one by one; the Wassermann reaction, the only one still standing, is currently the object of energetic attacks by the same people who made a living off it for years . . . There are frequent reports of syphilis cases that evolved silently, without producing positive serological reactions but abruptly revealing themselves through tertiary clinical symptoms." Demonic possession and divine grace proceed in the same fashion . . .

He is right to talk about "the terrifying cave of our etiological ignorance," but this dark cave is the only thing that can really attract a sharp, disinterested mind to the study of medicine. Causes are a physician's horizon. He warns against too many analyses, too many blood samples, too many lumbar injections (too many X-rays, we should add): "Any introduction of extraneous substances into the circulation leaves residues of humors, with their attendant idiosyncrasies, hypersensitivities, and rejections; it modifies our individuality and our degree of humoral stability." He further remarks that "it is especially dangerous to place an instrument of physics in a doctor's hands: the more precise the instrument, the more certain we can be that from its measurements doctors will derive aberrant conclusions, discrediting the method of physics."

Fifty years ago the physician started to become a foot soldier; today he is a locomotive engineer, a bomber pilot. The state of our health probably depends on whether he luckily misses his target.

•

For Littré, *panser* is the same as *penser*, because if you wish to *panser* (to medicate, to heal), first you have to think. Then, as Paré used to say, God will do the healing.

•

One proof of physiologists' ignorance is their refusal to consider the mouth a sexual organ.

•

Ginger tea fortifies inner vision, expands the abilities of the buried eye, and makes the spirit whom it enters say: I can.

•

Mendacity is nature and truth artifice. To seek the truth is the goal of whoever looks behind the veil and goes against Nature, which does not wish to be seen in its nudity or intimacy—endless complication. No one is simple, no one at all. The more *simple* human beings are, the more they love the manure of mendacity, the more one has to lie to them, pretend to be simple while constructing an artifice. Without conventional lies, it wouldn't be possible to communicate with *simple* people.

•

No tomcat, however crazed with love, would purr at a female whose fur was saturated with the smell of smoke or who had blown a few puffs his way; but degenerate man allows his lovers to smoke.

.

A thread of invisible secretion, moved by a thought that barely grazes the soul, already contains an entire love story. For women, who experience loves made up of these irrelevant moments and feel no need to go any deeper, there is never solitude.

.

One of the ills caused by artificially prolonging life is that many people who wish to put an end to their days are forced to postpone the liberating act because they cannot inflict the pain of their suicide on their *elders*, who are still alive.

.

According to Stenson Hooker, the violent, passionate man emits bright red rays, the great thinker emits bright blue rays, the man who leads a wicked, dissolute life emits dirty brown rays, and the sick man emits olive rays (*The Lancet*, November 1905). What has happened to the bright blue rays?

.

A true philosopher knows the human being as an aggregate but neglects the parts, without ignoring them. His interest lies in the indivisible whole, an emanation of the absolute. He is an anatomist who has renounced the scalpel to squeeze more reality out of contemplation.

.

A homeopathic thought from Claude Bernard: "The action and disorderly effects of medicinal substances are analogous to the action and effects of the pathogenic causes."

Man is more complicated than the fly, which devours all the excrement it can find. Excrement is what the coprophagous man seeks in the body and would receive from the body, a living part of the body he craves while groping through its darkest alchemical intimacy. (A teardrop trickles from the eye, down the face's gutters, and is collected in the lover's mouth, though he would never lap up a teardrop found on a kitchen table.) This is idolatry, no minor sin. It is an analytic madness. A small part looks huge, a piece of the body is devoured, the whole crumbles, and the offended soul cries, "I'm Everything!" But no mouth can swallow a whole body, and the impossibility of ingesting the whole, the ineffable *Unum*, foments the maniacal love for organs, parts, secretions, and excretions, and transforms eroticism into an eternal curse. Every lover has *preferences*. There is no substantial difference between someone who loves the eyes and someone who loves excrement, teardrops, or urine. The preference indicates the erotic folly; only the degree varies. The wise man renounces all possessions and dreams of his beloved's ideal integrity.

.

Wondrously, Verlaine says that he searched for *un peu d'ombre et d'odeur* in woman. Shadow and smell—the mildest, most delicate scents of Eros, the indispensable shelter from pain —already contain a denial of the whole and reveal a body covered with dividing lines. But the true human measure lies within this aureate fervor for *un peu d'ombre et d'odeur*. Who could want more? The man who kills because of his sexual manias: for him the whole lies in destruction. The philosopher who rejects the orifices, which are parts, so as not to tarnish the absolute image of a being. But if he is human, when he winds up in bed with a woman, he turns to her parts and traces the dividing lines on her body.

·

Does cancer enter us or do we, in falling ill, enter the revelation of the universal cancer?

·

Example of erotic decomposition: "Whenever he kissed a rosy-faced little baby, he felt like cutting off its cheeks with a razor" (Lautréamont, *Les Chants de Maldoror*, Canto I). A straight-edge razor flourishes in the hand, invisibly brandished by even the tenderest lovers (Lucretius' *abradere*), but in rushes the angel who stayed Abraham's arm and turned his downward thrust into a tender caress. In the silence of the room, you can hear a faint click.

·

LA BOURBE—Soft mud! The name of an old lying-in hospital in Paris. Behold Mother and Newborn Child, and the mud that fills the earth and its hospitals.

·

The deluge of butchered meats that falls daily on Western cities portends massacres, disease, collective madness, dejection, mental confusion, and befoulment. More unhealthy energy to course through heads in the dark. This is the plague of quails in the Tombs of Lust (Numbers 11).

·

Man dares to keep permitting himself acts of cruelty, when already he calmly and repeatedly commits the cruelest act of all: procreating, consigning creatures who do not exist and do not suffer pain to the horror of life.

Fear is a contagion. Alain observed that most dangers are not very frightening, unless we see them reflected in another person's face, when almost none of us can resist a feeling of sudden terror.

·

At the climax of his oratorical raptures Hitler ejaculated; this was the moment the Crowd was completely in his thrall. He performed a monstrous copulation, an incest unknown to the sacred laws. The Crowd was impregnated with demons, who came out of its belly in no time. This explains how one man could be the father of so much evil.

·

The leather that flagellates contains the sacred force of the slaughtered beast: the voluntary flagellant is a weak man who prescribes a tonic for himself. If the flagellation is done with a branch, the patient experiences the fertilizing and fortifying influence of vegetation.

·

A moderate necrophile can easily be satisfied in the bed of a frigid woman.

·

Hesiod is right to call fear and terror the *children of Venus*; they gave birth to infectious diseases.

·

Exanastasis means both evacuation of the body and resurrection. Because the body cannot be resurrected unless it evacuates all matter.

The Silence of the Body

It is better to die emptying oneself than filling oneself, better to die from starvation than from indigestion.

•

The more asepsis is perfected in clinics, the more horrendous the dirtying of our living environment, of the water needed to rid our homes of impurities.

•

A woman for whom he nursed a secret passion removed her hand as if it were a glove and hung it on a nail in a crumbling wall alongside other things—utensils, instruments of torture. The man kissed the hand, his eyes searching for the mutilated woman. In the distance she smiled at him.

•

Lavatory dialogue: "Looking for 10–14-year-old girl to make her come." Answer, in a childish scrawl: "How much will you give me?" (She realized that she is supposed to put on a show and expects to be paid for her orgasm.)

•

". . . and of the spectator that went there, the spectacle remained" (Bartoli, death of Pliny the Elder).

•

Are only the dead true vampires? Maldoror says that because he is not dead but alive he is not a vampire, though he adores sucking blood from adolescent throats. So many definitions to revise. John Haigh, in the chronicles of vampire crime in London, becomes an ordinary murderer once he has lost this distinction; and if Maldoror is not a vampire, he is merely a somewhat outrageous homosexual.

•

Fake Syphilis (apply it to the penis or the vulva, like an artificial mole). Remove it after testing whether the lover's affection can withstand everything, or leave it on if one's boyfriend or girlfriend is in the mood for some terrifying fellatio or cunnilingus.

•

Isaac Babel, *Red Cavalry*: "I can see the wounds of your god oozing seed, a fragrant poison to intoxicate virgins." As if Catherine of Siena were walking amid the Cossacks in a dream.

•

Cesare Serono observed that chemical substances, like various forms of radiation, are determining causes of tumors and not merely predispositional causes (*Rassegna di clinica, terapia e scienza*, 1947). He classified the abuse of artificial vitamins and of synthetic sex hormones with the most active predispositional causes, while he attributed the increase of cancer in the countryside to anticryptogamians with an arsenic base. His allusion to the carcinogenic action of aerial power lines suggests the image of a net, of the web in which we live, awaiting the Great Spider: "We live beneath an electric net that subjects us to the influence of obscure discharges affecting our organic metabolism."

•

Life yearns, in secret, to cease to exist. Sometimes it even shouts it, but we do not hear.

•

Today women have their doctors; yesterday they had their confessors. The modern confessors will cause no fewer disasters than the old doctors did.

.

Laignel Lavastine and Vinchon, *Les Malades de l'Esprit et Leurs Médecins du XVI au XIX Siècle*, on the Bicêtre asylum during the French Revolution: The mystics were among the most dangerous inmates. The religious maniacs were exasperated and saddened by the disappearance of crosses and all cult objects, images, and the like, replaced—out of revolutionary idiocy—by tricolor cockades. Some committed suicide. For Christmas, one mystic planned to slit the throats of all the guards and all the other inmates; he managed to kill two people and wound a third. The mad reacted better than the sane, who accepted the change of symbols without protest—they even allowed the imposition of the new calendar and the new cults. But it is sad that extreme fidelity to signs not yet devoid of divine transmission should be manifested above all in the profound places of Madness. Quite a conflict remains: those forsaken by reason versus those imprisoned by Reason. The cockades bombard the crosses, which archaically respond with knife and cobbler's awl. "And God elected the follies of the world to cover the wise with shame." In this case he elected the cockade, since the cross had become too sapiential a symbol; the cross's defense was taken up by the Madmen at Dr. Pinel's Thermopylae. Thirty years later Esquirol would notice that *Mélancolie dévote* had almost disappeared, cured by tolerance. Crosses and cockades would coexist without hurting each other, and God continues to elect new forms of madness to shame the wise.

.

The Bicêtre inmates couldn't have been all that crazy. They hurled insults and threats at Couthon, the infamous paralytic who had come, in search of suspects, to sniff them out.

.

In *Des maladies mentales considerées* (1838), Esquirol says that almost all those who escaped the revolutionary scythe were afflicted by mental derangement.

.

Even the poorest and most squalid life is an Aeschylean drama, if you think of the tragedy of the bodily functions, the whispering of the secretions, the silence of the organs, the exertions of memory, the groping of the voice, the blood that courses, the mortal miasmas, the riots among microorganisms, the spermatic wars, the cellular eruptions, the pestilences of the nerves, the biochemical predestinations, and the fate that slowly but surely introduces you to the final infection, to the sores, the exploded boils, the snakes of madness, the furious bitches of Hunger.

.

"Those who glow because of their lively intelligence are often affected by epilepsy" (Johann Schenk of Grafenberg, 1520–98).

.

Dr. Benedetti writes about a *melancholic* and amenorrheic woman who left her house one night, naked, and went to a brothel, where she let herself be taken fifteen times. Afterward her periods returned, and she completely recovered from Melancholia.

.

The Silence of the Body

We are hovels and ratholes, inhabited by an occult face that bears no resemblance to us.

.

The gloomy sacred beauty of Augustine's portrait of St. Ambrose reading in silence in the *Confessions*: "His eyes scanned the pages and his mind explored the concept, while his voice was silent and his tongue was still" (VI,3). Augustine and other disciples entered and sat down in silence, trying to comprehend the strangeness of a *mental reading*. "But whatever he may have meant by this behavior, in such a man it could only be good." When we take our leave of the saint's quiet reading, we remain perplexed by his behavior: at that time, reading was only done aloud. Jackson Knight comments that the episode took place in the fourth century and constitutes a subject of immense importance since it mentions sound and pronunciation in ancient literary works. Poetry could not be poetry, he says, unless it was read aloud. Today a man who read verse or spiritual texts aloud while he was alone would be considered deranged. But St. Ambrose was accustomed to musical reading and certainly populated his silence with sounds without losing the voice of the text. He made himself imperceptible only to others.

.

"Lycanthropes have pale faces, dry eyes sunken within their heads, weak eyesight, with ne'er a teardrop, parched tongues, a strange thirst, and an extreme scarcity of saliva" (Tommaso Garzoni, *L'hospedale de passi incurabili*, 1594).

.

After the Black Death in the fourteenth century, fertility boomed and there were many twin births. None of these children had a full set of teeth: Nature, forced to be extremely lavish, neglected the details. Schopenhauer took this information from Schnurre's *Chronicle of the Epidemics.* The children of the survivors must have thought that man was an animal with fifteen or twenty-five teeth and that before 1340 only prehistoric man had thirty-two.

·

Perhaps owing to the sulphur that the intestines contain and blow out, sulphur has been regarded as an emanation of the Devil and the characteristic smell of the Inferno.

·

Fanny Targioni Tozzetti, old and decrepit, to a little girl who asked her why she had not requited the love of a poet like Leopardi: "My dear girl, he reeked."

·

Some American insurance companies grant special rates to clients who use homeopathic remedies, because they live longer.

·

The late-sixteenth-century physiologist Santorio recommended a special device for administering a clyster with one's own urine at its natural warmth, in order to stimulate peristaltic movement. The device is a bladder with an anal cannula, into which one urinates a moment before inserting the cannula. Too easy. Let us picture instead a catheter that carries the urine directly from the bladder to the rectum, transforming itself along the way from catheter to clyster, the Cathetolyster: the living image of an Ouroborus Snake, a uroproctological En-To Pan, profound Gnostic and alchemical symbol.

·

Erotomania is a word coined by Esquirol, who defines it in *Des maladies mentales considerées*: "Erotomania differs fundamentally from nymphomania and satyriasis. In the latter, the ailment originates in the reproductive organs, whose irritation affects the brain. In erotomania, love is in the head. Nymphomaniacs and satyromaniacs are victims of a physical disorder. Erotomaniacs are prey to their own imaginations."

.

Benjamin Ball, *La Folie érotique* (1888): A veteran of the Franco-Prussian War, a Latin teacher in a private school, chaste ("Most erotomaniacs are absolutely chaste"), is attracted exclusively by female eyes. He sees the cunt in the nostrils. He would like a girl with huge eyes for a wife . . . He seems like a lover of divine figures and archetypes; in its blindness the world provides him with a lunatic asylum as an altar. A seminarian thinks he has a hole in his skull through which the others (his fellow madmen) ejaculate their sperm into his brain. He says that when he sits down at the table, his nose, mouth, and intestines are full of sperm. He thinks he is everybody's prostitute. Another man had his chest devoured during coitus by a very lascivious woman: he is still alive but between his neck and his stomach there is a void, a huge hole covered by his suit. Ball tells malicious anticlerical stories, for instance that certain priests are in the habit of violating the corpses of people to whom they have given the last rites.

.

Mamtzer benidah (Made in Menstruation) is a terrible Hebrew insult. The Talmudists say that a *mamtzer benidah* is destined to vice and disease, a drunkard, madman, epileptic, murderer, cretin. Nothing can save him. But who has ever been *mamtzer benidah*?

Pregnant Athenians used to eat a lot of cabbage so the unborn child would be more vigorous. Hence the legend of babies born under cabbage leaves.

•

We have seen many seers among the blind: might not Cecum, the large intestine's monocle, be the profound seer of the body? Perhaps it issues warnings or omens that only the bowels understand, oracles intercepted by ears buried in the organic cosmos.

•

The Divine Comedy as an allegory of Digestion. The Mouth to the food: "Abandon all hope." Devils, Malebolge (stomach, "evil pouch," significantly called "evil," intestine); "round hole . . . to see the stars again" (anus). *Purgatory:* the assimilated substance remains in the body to suffer. *Paradise:* the voyage through matter has ended, that which was of Light has returned to Light, while for other foods the calvary recommences.

•

René Guénon said that archaeological digs, usually undertaken by professors incapable of understanding the profound meaning of certain ruins, can resuscitate tenebrous psychic forces that are irritated by purely material knowledge.

•

Guénon also said that in hands inadequately protected from the invasion of nether psychic forces, Tarot cards can become a dangerous instrument. Today all hands that toy with the Tarot are dangerous.

If today's ecological modifications are caused by malignant psychic forces acting in our world (in our sphere), fighting them with crude material means (imbecilic sophism: *good* versus *bad* Technology) can only provoke their scorn, because they are perfectly indifferent to material and practical means. The only thing that could force them to retreat would be a total shattering of the dominant fixed idea, a consequence of some unthinkable preaching, a conversion, a *teshuvah*, that, moving along mute paths, strikes out against the obscure currents and rips the gigantic weave of threads. An alternative is the protection of a certain number of Righteous Men who are very powerful, aware of the fact, and busy warding off the blow. Our poor *ecologists* have to content themselves with saving three or four trees, while in one fell swoop the demons knock down three hundred thousand trees across the world.

·

A noble idealist says: "The adolescent potentially represents a fundamental part of the force that must counter the technological ideal" (Dr. Gérard Mandel, *La Crise des générations*). Adolescents who save . . . Scarcely any of them will be saved.

·

The English psychologist Kenneth Strongman says that when two people stare at each other, the one who looks away first is the dominator. This may be true, because the stronger person is afraid of causing harm by staring too long, obscurely aware of the force and the powers of the eye and of the weak defenses of the person sitting opposite: but only people with a superior moral sense look away (which is partly what makes them dominators); the wicked, feeling strong, will never be the first to do so.

•

Voice heard in a dream:

If you wish the Temple's Veil to raise
Then search for Heaven's ancient gates.

I am on a street in Turin, one of my old streets. I enter a dimly lit corridor lined with old doors, locked, each one affixed with the Seal of Solomon, like a nameplate. (By *Temple* I mean the Templar Order.) Behind the last door I hear the voice of Elémire Zolla, who is examining a group of pupils.

•

If children mistreat an animal, even a big one, you must give them a spanking, because they are stronger and naughtier than the animal.

•

In the Canavese region (Piedmont), *tormenting Masses* were offered to bring harm to one of the living.

•

The further into the tragic we enter, the more our sense of the tragic diminishes. The role of the *fool* becomes prominent. And the Laughing Madman is the tragic in disguise, its last avatar, furnished with a safe conduct. Sophocles is missing, but there are thousands of black humorists.

•

"The first stage in the corruption of morals is the banishing of the truth . . . Our truth nowadays is not what is, but what we can persuade others to believe" (Montaigne, "Of Giving the Lie"). Yet morals seemed less corrupt in the very nations (U.S.S.R., China) where the truth was most tortured, slashed, dilapidated, and driven out. The reason was their poverty, for it ensured a certain cleansing of mores, counterbalancing the catastrophic effects of the impostors who ruled.

.

Before people who have been vaccinated against polio become prostatic and arteriosclerotic, the whole world might stop having toothaches.

.

The hydra of Les*bos* rather than Ler*nia*. A simple typographic error can annul a myth and replace it with a moral.

.

Madame Rochefoucauld says that cruelty is mother to kidney stones (in cruel people, I hope, and not in their victims).

.

A civilization boasted that it had discovered and reclaimed the sanctity of the body. Did it then honor this rediscovered and reclaimed sanctity? No, the civilization was happy with a simple written canonization in thousands of newspaper articles and books. Into the saint's face it threw chlorine, radioactive strontium, napalm.

.

Excrement is accepted as long as it is inside the body: it is not separated from the microcosm's unity. In isolation, excrement shocks and repels because it gives off the smell of denuded, anonymous soul.

.

41

In Chapter 7 of the second book of Maccabees, a mother tells her son, who is about to be sacrificed by Antiochus, that she nursed him for three years. Thus she exacerbates his martyrdom.

.

The smelliest parts of the body are those where more soul is collected. The eye, which is odorless, is *mirror* not soul. Adding perfume to the body adds soul or allows people with no soul to pretend to have one. The strongest smells have come to disgust us, because the more civilization represses and restrains natural animality, the more intolerable excessive soul becomes.

.

Rabbis allowed a Christian wizard to treat a sick Jewish man with the names of Jesus and the saints, because "the healing is brought about by the sound of the voice and not by the meaning of the words." The mystery of poetry is partly contained in this explanation. Poetry cannot be separated from its sound, otherwise it loses its therapeutic, prophylactic, and magic powers, its main components. If a translation into another language does not possess its own healing *sound*, it merely hints at the spell that can be cast by the original text.

.

A disease that obstructs evacuation is worse than one that obstructs satiation.

.

Two Babylonian tablets prescribe a cure for madness: Burn the madman at the stake or bury him alive. Suddenly insane asylums and electroshock sound compassionate.

The Silence of the Body

Ignorance about disease left more room for religious consolation and moral reflection. Knowledge of an infinity of causes and infectious processes (if we really do know them), rather than of the mystery of disease, has erased almost everything that made man *superior* to his afflictions. Imagination and moral force have been suffocated by the half-baked knowledge of medicine, the great corrosive, the depressing spirit. Here we are, forsaken, with neither invincible words nor small or large invocations, neither a reviving *Allah akbar!* nor Dreyer's *Ordet*, neither the moral Seneca nor our own enigmatic search for metaphysical solution. We are in the hands of medical technicians, who are more frightening than the disease, because they are inferior to it. They cannot understand pain; they shower tons of pharmaceutical TNT over a scrawny enemy armed only with clubs and imagine they are the victors.

·

It is painful to discover that a doctor is not God, because we cannot abandon the idea of a friendly, healing God above us.

·

The idea of a God causing one's destruction is a sublime etiology, raising man above his bed of torture and making him divine in his moment of greatest misery. "Neither does a God afflict you, nor does any God then heal you." Thus the only thing above this hospital ward is the upper floor, and above that another floor, and above still other floors, white and illuminated, and above me nothing more than a series of white illuminated floors criss-crossed by stretchers, where needles and scissors, gauze and thermometers are moving, and human hands grasp and let go of human hands. In the cellar a row of coffins, refrigeration cells: an aseptic, infinite, hopeless inferno.

.

A plastic surgeon from Padua, studying a relic from the fourth century of our era, an arm of St. Vincent the martyr, confirms that Vincent underwent torture by fire and died from the septicemia that subsequently arose.

.

A tribe of troglodytes in the Philippines wears an orchid over the pubis to ward off sterility. The fig leaf in Genesis covers nudity to protect it from the evil spirits that will assail mankind after sin.

.

The difference between North and South: "A wretch in the snow still has a social value, while a wretch in the sunlight is already putrefying" (Pierre MacOrlan, *Le Quai des Brumes*).

.

The Talmudists taught that certain demons dwell in lavatories. Including those at a Catholic university, where someone, still unknown, killed a girl with thirty-three stab wounds (Milan, July 1971). Those who committed crimes in these places could be acquitted, since they had been forced to kill by lavatory demons. Thus lawyers could also use demonology to paralyze criminal law. Beware if there is no Attendant! Often the attendant is a poor old woman, but strength does not matter: by virtue of being an attendant she is a living exorcism, a being that is neutral, refractory, unassailable by demons. The coins we give to a Public Restroom Attendant are compensation for his or her apotropaic activity, an offering

The Silence of the Body

to the protecting hands, which the vulgar think of as mere distributors of toilet paper.

•

A case of unrestrained omnivorism: Perrault's wolf, who indiscriminately gobbles up little girls and old women. He is not a true *werewolf* (humanoid) but rather a blind shark.

•

Russia tried to dominate us as a people and to convert us to its dogma; China hated us as former white masters. Which of the two potentates posed the worse threat?

•

Totapuri, Ramakrishna's Vedanta master, tries to drown himself in the Ganges because he can no longer bear the dysentery tormenting him; then the Devi appears to him, and he sees that the Devi is in all things and that all things are the Devi, even his dysentery. After emerging from the sacred waters that rejected him, he immerses himself in meditation. If it is true that during his respiratory attacks, Spinoza murmured, "My God, have pity on me, a sinner," then his heroic, human invocation was addressed to the respiratory attack.

•

Marriage without religious rites is a war that has been won. Now you can fight the war over again and lose.

•

An acrobat with curly brown hair and very dark skin performs difficult exercises on a trapeze suspended in mid-air. Very elegant and self-confident. After many revolutions, he serenely throws himself into the air, plummeting down into a green pool flickering with flames. (Maya. The hard part is throwing yourself. Once you have overcome the fear of diving, you are certain to find light and peace.)

.

A healer from Turin lived with a syphilitic woman and assures us he never got infected: *If there is love* there is no contagion. The explanation may not be convincing but it's nice.

.

Horace had bad eyesight (*lippus*), Virgil had bad digestion (*crudus*). (But Horace did not have a good stomach either.) Hermann Broch says the dying Virgil was a Clairvoyant Plant: his bad stomach was gone (*The Death of Virgil*). Becoming a plant is nicer than spreading the smell of sanctity in death.

.

It sounds like an item from today's news. Buddha died from poisoned mushrooms that he ate in the woods of a goldsmith. The Mushroom did not become the Buddhists' Crucifix; yet curiously, it is shaped like a Tau, a cross.

.

To keep us from seeing in the active forces of destruction the God whom we seek and love, a fiction like Satan is extremely convenient, for it screens the unbearable truth.

.

Mozart's passion for scatology, eroticism, dirty language, verbal crudeness . . . He had black reserves, his own Inferno of impure sounds that he transformed into Edenic plenitude inside the Angelic Chamber: his *nigredo* and *albedo*.

.

The Silence of the Body

In despair, they look to the doctor as a shaman or holy man: the frightened, obtuse doctor barricades himself behind Technology, Chemistry, Physics, Experiments, Analysis.

·

From a description of Parkinson's disease: "The face is often fixed and rigid, and when the patient hints at a smile, he or she does so in a persistent manner." Nothing should last longer than the second required by its need to exist: a smile that persists instantly becomes a lugubrious grimace. All pointless perdurance, even without rigidity or trembling, is Parkinson's.

·

Aleister Crowley told the doctor who would not give him morphine in his agony that for refusing him the morphine the doctor would follow him into death. The doctor did not have the time to refuse morphine to others.

·

Haarmann, the butcher of Hanover (thirty known murders: children lured into his house, sodomized, cut into pieces, the flesh sold on the black market during the economic crisis), decapitated in 1925, wanted a tomb with this epigraph: Hier ruht der Massenmörder—Here rests the mass murderer. This is a unique association of the ordinary *ruhen* with the original *Massenmörder*. If they had let him have his way, the epitaph "mass murderer" would have punished him more than the executioner's ax: it would have pointed him out to his victims' *Manes*, and forbidden rest for the mass murderer.

·

A Yiddish proverb: "Beware of silent water, a silent dog, and a silent enemy."

47

•

Bartolini, *De insolitis partus humani viis* (1664): The *insolitis viis*, unusual ways, include a Spanish maid's expulsion of a child from her mouth. Witkowski says these cases can be explained by the growth of the fetus outside the uterus and its expulsion *par les voies supérieures* after it perforates the wall of the stomach (*Histoire des accouchements*). Other interesting cases: fetuses that come out of the navel, the hypochondrium, the hips, the anus, and the bladder. Witkowski claims the first cesarean section on a living woman was performed in 1500 by a certain Nufer, a pig castrater from a village in Thurgau, on his wife, Elizabeth Alespachin: "The woman was laid on a table, her husband made an incision in the abdomen, as if he were working on a pig, and on the first try pulled out the child." Better yet: a cesarean performed by having a bull pierce the woman's belly with its horns. This is recorded in a painting in the Saardam church (Holland).

•

Andrea Doria said he could not die, since he had never been born (he was born by cesarean section). Macbeth's murderer, Macduff, is not *born of woman*, and when he stabs Macbeth he reveals to him that he was born by cesarean section. We have lost a profound idea: Slit abdomen is not woman, there is man but there is no *birth*, the *unborn* man will be invulnerable, perhaps immortal. The *cunnus* is the sign of a woman, and if you are not born from there, where the woman dwells, the *mother* (the uterus) who bore you is neither your mother nor of your mother. Since cesarean section has become common practice, soon more of us will be *unborn* than born. Nature had no problem tolerating the exception, but what about the rule (or almost the rule)? Cesarean children also say *my mother*, but something is definitely less filial and less maternal in their lives.

The Silence of the Body

·

It happened in Belfast. There are some men who would go so far as to shoot at a one-and-a-half-year-old girl from a moving car, out of a generic *political* hatred for the people in her neighborhood. The gunman, no doubt, considers himself a *combatant*.

·

Do faces belong to the body? Sometimes I have my doubts. They seem to lead independent lives, meeting each other unburdened by the rest of the body. Faces come directly from the demonic and from the angelic, from the depths and from the heights; the rest is merely terrestrial.

·

We throw everything into these poor vessels—all the soul's excretions, all the mind's diseases, all the blackness of life —and we call it *love*. And if this poison of ours does not turn into a being that resembles us, we feel imperfect, mortal, helpless.

·

There is solace and strength in the thought that some books can liberate and save us. We add new books to our collection almost every day, but the ones we need have already been around for some time.

·

Philosophy, says Montaigne, is nothing more than sophisticated poetry, and Plato an incoherent poet. Littré defines *sophistiquée* as *subtilisée avec excès*.

·

Carbon monoxide wishes you a good morning, carbon monoxide wishes you a good night. It feeds you, follows you, accompanies you, sleeps, walks, and wakes with you. It is always around you, always near, always on your breath. Carbon Monoxide, what is your true name in the legions of Abaddon?

·

An emancipated woman is much less frightening than a subjugated woman. I suspect that the enemies of women's liberation are secretly in love with what is evil in woman: the accursed fire that flares from her under the anvil of servitude.

·

A man acclaimed is a man enchained.

·

The most difficult maxim to follow is the *Pirkei Avot*'s "Do not look down on anyone."

·

Georges Bernanos, in a letter to Henri Massis: "I think that our children will make up the bulk of the Church's troops on the side of the forces of death. I will be shot by Bolshevik priests with the *Social Contract* in their pockets and the cross on their chests." The revolutionary priest on the firing squad is more priest than ever: after much useless sloth he retrieves the sacred insignia and begins to sacrifice. He is performing his role. Beware of him! See the figure of Cimourdan in Victor Hugo's *Ninety-three*.

·

PIG, THE BACON MACHINE (*Corriere della Sera*). Only five kilograms per capita in Italy; forty in Germany. Come on,

Italy! Develop your jaws. *Bacon pig*. People who use expressions like this, and newspapers that allow them, are spreading the evil omen of obscenity. The poor offended bacon will take its revenge.

·

With great humanity, Chamfort explains something I have asked myself many times: Why do people have children under intolerable political regimes? "Because nature has laws that are gentler, but more imperious, than those of tyrants; because children smile at their mothers under Domitian the same way they did under Titus." Vittorio Alfieri addresses this issue in *On Tyranny*. "I conclude: that a man who has a wife and children under tyranny is repeatedly enslaved and humiliated as many times as there are individuals for whom he is forever forced to tremble (I, 14)."

·

The profession of listening to many forms of howling and wailing teaches a person to mercifully offer an open garment —the mouth—to the wretched nudities that come running.

·

Scenes of souls being slaughtered are always illuminated. The massacre started long before the hours began to rush by and will continue even after their sound has ceased.

·

Problems of overpopulation. "If everyone were to use leaves from trees to wipe their ass, in no time at all the remaining trees would have no leaves." "Then we'll have to use our fingers, like in prehistoric times." "Yes, but we won't be able to wash our fingers because of the water shortage. After too much use, we'll have to cut them off." "The most powerful countries will order the weakest countries not to wipe at all, on pain of extermination by the Death Ray."

.

The *waste* land, bereft of human beings; only humanity's love for itself can imagine the earth on the verge of devastation. In reality, the earth is devastated that it is not a wasteland. Unfortunately, *we* will never know the profound delight felt by a true wasteland.

.

A beautiful thought from Le Clézio: "Perhaps one day we will realize there was no art but only Medicine."

.

The difference between a Sadist and a Perfect Catharist is that the latter tries not to imitate the horror he has understood but to drive it from himself and diminish its deadly effects around him.

.

The future's inhumanity makes it possible to predict its impossibility. Once a certain degree of inhumanity has been reached, which we are fairly close to, nothing more can happen to man because man will no longer exist. The non-man who might be able to withstand inhuman excesses does not interest the man we still are.

.

According to Aleister Crowley, on March 21, 1904, after the eon of Isis and the eon of Osiris, the world entered the eon of Horus, God of Ecstasy and of Violence, and above all the God of Fire. Nearly a century of the new eon has gone by: the human world is a burning island surrounded by a sea of fire. Some Righteous Men are delaying the fire's action by keeping watch and praying, as are, perhaps, the surviving written words, and the desperate force inside trees, which are sacred to the gods above.

The figures of horrifying demons have already passed by —Lenin, Hitler, Stalin, and the scientists who freed the atom—and postwar reconstruction was another face of Destruction. Metal, the earth's chthonic fruit, is another fire; mineral oil, the ancient Greek fire, chokes the waters surrounding the emerged lands. But I would begin the eon of fire one year earlier, with that miserable congress of Russian émigrés, in a London polluted by coal, great Hubris of stone and metals. There the furies converged on Ulyanov's will, and amid the pandemonium, the serpent of the Leninist fraction emerged. In that year, even Kaiser Wilhelm II, that idiot, seems to have been working toward the triumph of the man of destiny.

.

Charles Du Bos observed that Dostoevsky's psychological descriptions presuppose direct cooperation with Satan.

.

In a Parisian clinic, Ernst Jünger saw ninety-two-year-old twin sisters who had simultaneously developed cancers in their breasts (or in the spots where their breasts used to be).

.

On December 9, 1971, in Paris, a twenty-three-year-old teacher, Jean Siche, killed himself with gas. The gas's composition: the student uprising combined with his colleagues' lack of solidarity.

.

Desecration is easy work; hence it should repel us.

.

Collages give you the pleasure of cutting up human beings
—individuals and crowds—without shedding a drop of blood.
They are the best surrogate for crime. The spirit of Destruction is released, satisfied, and what remains is pleasing to the
eyes, odorless, and can be saved or sold.

.

On the night of December 30, 1971, a soul in pain was
moaning inside the Assisi fortress.

.

Living in dread of mankind. With the disappearance of ferocious animals and the removal of the sky's terrors—pleasant
distractions by comparison—the only remaining source of fear
is man. The cities have turned into organizations of fears,
immense fortresses of man's fear of man. Inside the cities,
socializing takes on the form of feudal self-defense, an uncontrollable spread of mutual distrust. A postal worker is
separated from the person asking for a stamp by bulletproof
glass that can withstand a bomb. The Terror State provides
the best protection against individual crime; it performs
psychectomy and nousectomy on all the citizens it protects.
Outside the gates: man, the abyss into which we fall.

.

How can we consider those who are most terrified by the
human face abnormal and mentally ill? The true madness is
not to fear it, not to be ashamed of it, given the things of
which it is capable. The terrifying sensation of being surrounded, besieged by man, knowing that from one moment
to the next the law, all moral restraints, can snap, blow,

The Silence of the Body

explode; at times, the law seems to be sustained only by a miracle or a momentary calm. Earthquakes, which have never ceased to race through the earth in all directions, provide a kind of relief for man's diseased cities (finally a different fear! a fear without a human face!). I think of the wolves at the beginning of François Villon's *Petit testament*, driven into Paris during the *morte saison*. Wolves of an extinct hunger and cold, their howling heard fearfully from behind bolted doors—my heart is moved by the thought.

•

Walking through the countryside today is like visiting an old neighborhood that is being demolished.

•

"But poetic meter is incorruptible: its invisible columns and portals cannot be touched by the flames of destruction" (Ernst Jünger, *On the Marble Cliffs*). I think so too. Back to work.

•

At Fort Collins there is a germ plasm bank of plant seeds from all over the world, because plant life is disappearing and some people think that in a few years the germ plasm that has not been collected in banks will be lost forever. Everything has become bank, museum, archive; everything that we call life is already in glass cases. Who are the visitors and customers? The formerly living, the literal *Refaim*, the Weak. Only dead souls, set dancing by an electric wire, still desire this state of nonliving—already the norm for many—so they can visit the Museum of Life during regular hours.

•

A delegation from Milan visits Bethlehem, the site of ancient prophecies, it would seem. The mayor of Milan relates: "In

Bethlehem I asked the Franciscans and the mayor of the city if I could do something for them. The friars and the Arab mayor replied that I should look into having a Fiat agency opened as soon as possible" (January 11, 1972).

•

A room lit by extremely high lamps. From a group of naked women, one, whom he had met many years earlier, broke away and invited him to whip her, offering him a two-tailed whip. While rhythmically whipping her, he thought how delicious flagellation was, and her full satisfaction proved it to him. Then she lay down on a table, begging him not to stop; her ass, when he kissed it, was as hollow as a drum. Later, entering a little Nordic house at dawn, he found two little girls in bed and affectionately hugged them; then he entered the room of their mother, who did not seem like a stranger to him, and kissed her deeply slumbering face. He lay on top of her with great yearning and pleasure, and the woman showed how happy she was to see him. The two faces of Eros in a single night: cruelty and the theft of delicate love, infernal rapture and celestial abandon.

•

An old doctor says, "Health is a precarious state for man that bodes no good."

•

Christ, you are the one true drug! This is how he is invoked by the drug addicts of the Jesus movement in California. They cannot imagine how right they are, as proven by two thousand years of human history.

•

The destruction of poetry begins in the idea of language as pure convention, an aggregate of signs, the result of a game of chance, like the cell. No one who thinks of language this way could still believe in the power of words ordered within the architecture of *carmen*, in the good that words must emanate once they have become a versified lump, a musical apparition, capable of revealing something of the hidden God, creator of letters, whose rhythm and sense carve the forbidden figure and trace the ineffable Name.

·

Sophocles' Philoctetes says that his illness returns after many days, "when it is tired of running around elsewhere." *Nosos*, illness, is a ferocious beast that breaks away from us for a time and roams the countryside. Disease never rests, biting others while we catch our breath, until it returns and starts again. Maybe it has its own clock.

·

Morbus sacer, holy illness, is what Apuleius called epilepsy in the *Apology*, because it afflicts the brain, the most sacred part of man. But his explanation is Hippocratic secularization (*De morbo sacer* denies that the gods cause our illnesses). Before Hippocrates, antiquity considered every disease sacred because of its divine origin. Disease was a divine affliction; collapsing and foaming at the mouth were signs of an even greater divine possession: the holiest illness of all, oracular disease. But in Latin, epilepsy was also called *morbus comitialis* (an evil omen if it occurred at the *comitia*, the election assembly), which removes any trace of the sacred. There were mysterious cures: Eat the meat of an animal whose throat was slit with a knife that had killed a man or partake of a goat roasted on a funeral pyre; drink the blood of a slain gladiator.

·

A long cigarette butt squashed out in a toilet bowl is like a man's moral portrait. There he is: vulgar, overbearing, stupid, ungenerous, all for himself in coitus, loaded with dirty or stolen money, indifferent to other people's tragedies, destroyer of animals and plants, hunter, sports-page reader, greedy, overbearing in everything, noisy, loud-mouthed, crassly practical, red-meat eater, salt shaker, coffee drinker, dressed in expensive suits, perfumed, respecter of power, and car lover. When he went to take a piss, he left his picture; his name doesn't matter.

·

Karl Jaspers to Rudolf Bultmann: "By applying the methods of technology to actions and behavior that technology cannot dominate, scientific superstition leads to a specific, devastating activity, analogous to magic's aberrations, which have never been overcome."

·

I am going to copy in its entirety a stupendous thought of Joseph Joubert's, dated June 26, 1806: "Even hatred of evil can make men evil, if it is too strong, too dominant, too isolated (so to speak) from our other feelings. Hence our books have inspired evil, calling attention only to the tragedies associated with certain abuses. This is the source of the monstrous events we have witnessed. Violent lessons in humanity were followed by horrifying cruelties. Compassion became furor. We massacred Louis XVI, his sister, and all that was most virtuous in France, out of ferocious love for the American black and ferocious horror at the St. Bartholomew's Day Massacre. Too forceful and too frequent representations of human suffering have made hearts inhuman. Taking the pathetic to the extreme is a deadly source of callousness in men."

For two hundred years images of suffering have been thrust at crowds to unleash their ability to produce even worse images. The wars and revolutions of this century are mainly the result of tableaux of human suffering that were able to excite the most complete inhumanity. A picture seen in a newspaper one morning can conjure out of nowhere a fanatical leader of paid assassins. At least *L'Ami du Peuple* wasn't illustrated.

.

"Woman is tradition, just as man is progress; and without them there is no life" (Amiel, May 6, 1852). But what if woman wants to be *progress* too? The lack of an opposite direction, of a restraining force, leads to chaos and disaster. *Progressive* women contribute catastrophically to accelerating a movement initiated by man, and their revolts consist solely in the paranoia of propelling to victory *exactly* what man wants.

.

To a man from Medina who practiced magic against scorpions and asked Muhammed if it was lawful, the Prophet replied: "Whoever can be useful to his fellow man should be so."

.

Near Salerno, on February 25, 1972, a cow gave birth to a calf with six legs, a single eye in the middle of its head, and the snout of a rhinoceros. Twenty centuries ago this could have meant that Caesar would die. Today, if a cow gave birth to the Leviathan, it would still mean nothing (there are no more Caesars).

.

Nature is protected by holy interdict, not by good manners and not by civil law. If the olive tree is sacred to a god, the olive tree will not be cut down. If the pig is sacred, no one will eat it. But the holy interdicts that protected the Great Mother have disappeared, and a monotheism that is ever more monoatheistic has destroyed all the cults and sacred fears of nature. The earth is not sacred; it can be destroyed, as Spinoza predicted. In a complete vacuum of holy interdicts, the most devastating science has suddenly emerged and set about its business. How long, O Lord? As long as one olive tree is left standing, as long as there is still an owl in a tree, as long as there is still one molecule of water with a tiny bit of life in it.

•

"We poor doctors: none of our remedies has the wondrous power of a woman's hand placed over an aching forehead. At that decisive moment, science vanishes, and the anguish of a soul sinking into the boundless solitude of the beyond comes to rest on woman, full of the world" (Gregorio Marañon, *Soledad y libertad*). Consoling thought, but *full of the world* is a flash of revelation.

•

A Citroën abandoned on the side of a road. Compare it to *une charogne*, a dead body. You turn a corner and there, suddenly, is the dead car, the automobile carcass. You can see its decomposition, rust, dents, and exposed viscera. But there is no sound, no strange music of insects, and above all no smell. This is the almost metaphysical decomposition, more immaterial than material, of an automaton that lived, that felt *conatus* (effort) without ever acquiring human characteristics. It decomposes the way it lived, inhumanly.

•

Cancer, which used to live separately, has been summoned to become as big as the earth. If only we still knew how to sanctify!

The Silence of the Body

One of King Philip II's prisons was named after St. Theresa. In Moscow an oratorio was sung called *Lenin, Heart of the Earth*.

•

In Goethe's day, water consumption was 30 liters a day per capita. Today it is 200 liters; in the United States it reaches 450 liters. Between homes and industries, it gets as high as 1,500 liters. Runoff water from the mountains has grown scarce, while the fresh and salt waters on the surface are fatally ill; the oxygen exchange struggles to take place. In Europe, the Rhine carries the waste of thirty million people, along with an infernal quantity of industrial waste: the mouth of the Rhine is a gigantic chemical murderer. Under these conditions, can you still talk about the *future of society*?

•

A friend who has cancer told me what it's like to be alone with the machine that is radiating cobalt 60 over her chest. The machine talks: its strange humming gets louder one minute and stops the next. She lies there in complete isolation, with a heavy door behind her, while her ambiguous companion looms over her. It is known to be deadly, and everyone flees and fears it. With you alone it should show itself full of goodness and heal you in exchange for money. But what language does this monster speak? What warnings does it whisper? What stories does it tell? Perhaps it speaks of others who have come, now dead, and advises you not to fool yourself, honestly begs you: Do not think that I can defeat death.

•

"In life's human reality, the fight against pain is a form of usury, even for the great mystics. Assenting to pain is a slow suicide, because even when great sufferings are silent, they are never mute" (René Leriche, *Chirurgie de la douleur*).

.

The world bewitched. A massacre of unarmed people at an Israeli airport by *Japanese* gunmen is praised by the *Egyptian* government as an example of *Arab* courage.

.

More forcefully than Pascal, Carlo Emilio Gadda calls "I" the most lurid pronoun of all. Some example he sets.

.

I went into the house where the accountant N. had just died. His mother approached me in black, sobbing, and this puzzled me when I thought of how many times her son had savagely beaten her. The dead man was laid out in a room adorned like a church during Easter week, all gold and candles, and while his mother told me how suddenly her son had died, the rooms flowed together toward the windows like rivers. But there I sat like an outside observer, unable to fathom her excessive grief.

.

"The crimes of extreme civilization," says Barbey d'Aurevilly, "are certainly more atrocious than those of extreme barbarity." We are civilized to the extreme . . .

.

A psychiatrist on the Baader-Meinhof gang: "They seek salvation in a paranoia that blinds them to reality, because they believe everything that surrounds them is an evil machination." On this point they are not blind. Man cannot, however, look upon the underlying evil and thus cannot escape the punishment of total blindness and corruption meted out to all except inspired seers, and especially those athletes who have overcome evil and been immunized before approaching the vision. For Arjuna the sight of God in his terrifying aspect is cathartic; he remains a warrior and a righteous man. For a Baader, a glimpse behind the veil produces mental upheaval.

.

Thyroid and pain. Leriche observes that by increasing or decreasing the calcium dosage, the parathyroid glands interfere with the harmony of the nervous system and with the susceptibility to and hence the genesis of pain. Every nervous imbalance in an apparently normal life may be simply a distant reflection of a parathyroid game, of a slight hormonal disturbance, of karmic dust, or of Psyche's trembling.

.

Leriche attained the first of the four Buddhist truths, the first degree of *Samadhi*, the understanding of suffering, a great achievement for a Western doctor. But severing the nerves does not suppress pain, because it does not suppress *tanha*, which continuously produces pain, forcing us inside the circle: "Praeterea versamur ibidem atque insumus usque—We spend our lives in the same place and are there continually" (Lucretius, III, 1080).

.

"True doctors are few and little known, for almost all physicians are true invalids" (Giordano Bruno, *Ash Wednesday Supper*).

.

A normal calcium count is required to prevent pain in the joints. The adrenal substances are vasoconstrictive and cause pain (Leriche). Contemporary life seems deliberately designed to upset the calcium balance and continuously stimulate the adrenal glands; all it takes is a mechanical whistle to upset the nervous system, inducing vasoconstriction. The balance is restored by drugs, which in turn, after a certain period of use, produce imbalances. By altering the nervous system after temporarily suppressing pain, analgesics and anesthetics create another pain, more suited to the new sensibility.

.

With extraordinary subtlety, Leriche notes an individual privilege: "Not everyone may be capable of producing a painful syndrome." This is one way to restore karma and predestination.

.

An itchy groin can lead to suicide. To get rid of his, Marat waited for Charlotte to ring twice.

.

In the Chieri cathedral, amid a sea of faces, two rites take place simultaneously: on a big stage a Jewish ceremony with rabbis (one of whom is black) dressed in white, readings of the Torah, and the singing of Psalms; at the main altar a Catholic pontifical *missa solemnis*, with priests in full regalia, flowers, and organ music. The Jewish ceremony ends with dances and joyous outbursts, amid the crowd's applause. All at once, the crowd disappears; there are no more rabbis or priests; the church is deserted. The only person left is a short, greasy woman, an old cleaning woman perhaps, with long, limp hair and a cracked black patent-leather purse, descending the steps of the main altar. I turn to her for an explanation and the woman slips away, becoming smaller and smaller, and when she disappears a big cat with yellow spots takes her place, writhing around on the floor. The cat stares at me: it has yellow eyes, brimming with phosphorus, powerful. Ah, I shout, finally I understand: It's all your work, none of it was true, there is no possible reconciliation, I recognize you and I am not afraid of you. I confront the cat (but I'm not afraid of it) and it backs off, hissing. Then I back away from it, insulting it and desperately shouting that I am not afraid (June 19, 1972, in the morning).

•

Rosenbaum says that the rabbis derive *Baal-Peor* from בעד *(aperire: himinem virgineum*—"to open: the virginal hymen"). In Greek: *peos, peoidês,* that which has a swollen penis. Penis is from *peos,* not from *a pendendo,* because the parts of the body get their names in action rather than in repose. (But "arm" or "hand" describes neither action nor rest.) *Baal-Peor,* Lord of the Penis. *Bet-Peor,* House of the Penis, city of Peor. (See Numbers 25 and 31.)

Rosenbaum imagines that the Mosaic laws on sexual purity resulted from the venereal epidemic of Baal-Peor (*Histoire de la syphilis dans l'antiquité*). But then Moses becomes a doctor fighting an ordinary epidemic with somewhat bloody prophylactic procedures. If Moses is divested of his sacerdotal wisdom and prophetic mandate, he also loses his crowning achievement: constructing Order from man's violent disorder—the true, epic Prophylactic, because everything allied with the divine *tremendum* also wards off disease, the lightning of God. But the Alexandrine hypothesis, disputed by Josephus Flavius in *Against Apion,* already framed Exodus in an epidemic climate. Whether syphilis was in the daughters of Moab, in the Egyptian women already (which Guiart, Fournier, Ruffer, and Smith deny), or dwelling in Jacob's tents, from which Moses tried to expel it with extermination and the stake, is a purely ideological question, to be decided by anti- or philo-Semitism.

.

Aristotle says that the *pathicus*, the invert, is knock-kneed and has evil, shifty eyes, a head that leans to the right, limp wrists, and legs that cross when he walks. Polybius observes that his voice is flute-like, trembling, and shrill. Philo Judaeus invoked the death sentence (an essentially demographic measure) for those who suffered from *nousos thêluia* (the effeminate illness), because they spread sterility and impotence. In Sodom, cinaedopathy—the sin against nature—was hereditary. (Why destroy them with fire? Soon they would have been extinct.) Juvenal also sees cinaedopathy as a *morbus*, a disease: Peribomius gives away his illness *vultu incessuque*, "by his demeanor and by his walk" (II, 17).

.

The dying forest, where beautiful animals and birds disappear, is increasingly populated by snakes. The last shocking emblem of life outside of man is a multiplying of teeth with a poisonous bite.

.

The overly slow exchange of gases in conifers, strangled by oily layers of pollution, is laying waste to the vegetation in the Alpine valleys. The plague has also settled there, and in the woods of the Val d'Aosta we were passing through there were countless dying trees, pines destroyed by lichens and blighted junipers without a single berry. A tiny fragment of Shiva's dance over the cemetery of the world. The demons of vegetation at work: legions of parasites descend on green plants and devour them. The fir tree is the conifer with the best resistance: solitary green hero amid thousands of shameful pines with leper's bells dangling from their necks. A tree stripped of its branches and split, not by the ax, but solely by the vicinity of man and the breath of his devices. God is dead, the tree is dead, life above the tree is dead, life is dead.

·

Job and Philoctetes. Similar in their complaints, and probably also in their disease, cut short by divine epiphany (YHWH, Heracles), they differ in their sexual destinies. When Job is healed he returns to the joys of the family and fathers seventeen children, amid flocks of sheep and camels that breed. Philoctetes, whose nature has changed in the solitude of Lemnos (*Lemnia egestas*), is made permanently *mollis*, effeminate, by Aphrodite, *goel* of Paris' blood:

> *Mollis erat facilisque viris Poeantius heros:*
> *volnera sic Paridis dicitur ulta Venus.* *
> (Martial, II, 84)

According to the scholiast of Thucydides, Philoctetes could not bear his disgrace so he left his homeland and founded a city called Malachia (Softness, Languor), a type of Sodom. Malachia's derivation is Semitic: *malàtz*, to be soft. Wouldn't it be great if Philoctetes were the founder of Sodom! There is something equally unsatisfying in the easy moral of Job and in the complicated amorality of the Greeks, maybe because, after the tragic cry, neither the reward nor the punishment provides a resolution that is truly tragic.

·

Our poor lives as witnesses of the end. What can we do? Fast into silence, suicide, or submission.

---

* "The hero Poeantius was effeminate and yielding to men: they say this is how Venus avenged the wounds of Paris."

Aulus Gellius says that Socrates was saved from the Athenian plague by temperance, abstinence, and a regimented life, *ut nequaquam fuerit communi omnium cladi obnoxius*—so that he was in no way responsible for the common destruction of all. Beautiful myth, possible event. Temperance is the opposite of, the true antidote to, plague, which is disorder, confusion, coming undone, and losing control. But it is a classic allopathic cure. Homeopathy requires a temperance that is not too rigid: a dose of the plague, well diluted.

·

"So I pray to our sweet Saviour that he guide us to mangle and mortify our bodies" (Saint Catherine to Fra Tommaso della Fonte). What was Catherine doing in the Siena hospital? What only sublime doctors know how to do: letting herself be mangled by sick people.

·

Karl Kraus says that "diagnosis is a very widespread disease," because the Vienna school was more interested in diagnosing than in curing. You can only understand his aphorism by remembering the *therapeutic nihilism* of which the Vienna medical school stood accused.

·

Perfect adaptation to contemporary urban life is a sign of serious imbalance. Only those who suffer from city life are healthy. The signs of imbalance that result from conscious suffering and incompatibility are proof of sound mental health.

·

The body is perfid and treacherous: it is a Thug who travels with us. It smiles at life and is a killer sent by death.

•

The most dangerous weapon ever invented is man.

•

A minister explains to me that everyone's teeth should be pulled, one by one, to improve humankind. Naturally, dentures would be punishable by death. With its mouth empty, humanity becomes easier to educate, its harshness easier to soften, its voracity easier to tame.

•

There is a profound relationship between childbirth and the outhouse. A woman who wishes to hide her delivery locks herself in the outhouse and, in a tragic purgation, rids herself of the infant by throwing it down the hole. *Clamant latrinae latibula ubi sunt pueri suffocati*—The hiding places of the latrine, where the children were suffocated, cry out! Newborn man as dead excrement. Infanticide has become rare, perhaps because with the universal spread of the bathroom and the monitoring of public latrines, the authentic outhouse, fomenter of demons, is in decline.

•

"Every diversion is an anticipation of hell." Well said, José Bergamín, but terrible! These words were not spoken by a fanatical fifteenth-century preacher but by a brilliant contemporary writer. The *infernal* substance of diversion consists, I believe, in its literal meaning: to take another way.

•

"The influence of our political misfortunes has been so pervasive that I could recount the history of our revolution, from the storming of the Bastille to Bonaparte's last appearance, through the story of a few lunatics whose madness is tied to the events that have marked this long period in our history" (Esquirol, *Des maladies mentales considerées*).

·

In the *Mémoire historique et statistique sur la Maison royale de Charenton*, written in 1835, Esquirol recalls the plays that the *trop fameux* Sade staged between 1805 and 1811. His plays were not therapeutic psychodramas but teasing and abuse of the sick. I do not know if any of Sade's biographers has remarked that his nastiest deeds were the parties and shows he put on at Charenton in his final years, using weak, innocent people to entertain a crowd of Parisian idlers who ran to the madhouse looking for thrills. While Sade may not have deserved the Bastille for his disrespect to a "whore's ass," the Charenton parties earned him the well-deserved fate of never leaving the asylum. The only thing that came near little Magdeleine Leclerc was a jockstrap.

·

Villon exaggerates: the flames of love are neither hotter nor more deadly than *feu Saint Antoine*. Look at the Fire on Grünewald's altar and immediately you will say: Better the cruelest love.

·

Tattoos were all the rage among whores during the Napoleonic era. On their arms they bore the name of the man who exploited them, and on their bellies the name of their favorite woman. To the moralists who were striving to abolish slavery: behold an intrepid response from indomitable slaves.

The Silence of the Body

•

They were a beautiful couple. Her wealth of varicose veins matched his complete lack of teeth.

•

If it were not predestined, it would be an utterly absurd project to contemplate founding new states when in fifty years or so there will only be termites, mice, and deformed shadows creeping through huge deserted craters. All these newly founded states, born and bred in blindness, will participate in abetting that desolation.

•

Anne Boleyn had three breasts (one was inguinal) and six fingers on each hand. *Ne quid nimis*—nothing too much. Cutting off her head was a reparative Nemesis.

•

A Jewish woman said that she dreamed her cunt was called *ghetto*. Was she thinking about the separate neighborhood and its little shops? About the pogroms? About the fears?

•

Inland from Cagliari the big toes on many women are tapered. A mother will often let her baby suck on one to keep it quiet when her hands are busy. Sometimes she gets the baby drunk too.

•

In churches the pulpit is no longer used, because the priest is no longer supposed to stand above the faithful—he is an *equal*. But by descending from the pulpit, the priest ascended to stupidity; he did not become *equal* to the faithful. Before, he used to soar above the flock, in flight like a bat. He rose as high as the cupola, descended to touch the pews, turned turned turned, and filled the chapels and naves. The apotropaic pulpit warded off misery and stopped the demons that were flying toward him from the kneeling or distracted *massa luti* (mass of mud).

·

Opera seemed unchangeable, but today there is great airplane traffic behind the scenes. The Trovatores and Traviatas move through the air, the Flying Dutchmen really fly, the fat Aidas swoop down on the dressing rooms like hawks, the Queens of the Night fall from the sky, and a Barber of Seville flies at an altitude of twelve thousand meters toward Tokyo, taking the polar route.

·

A survivor of Mauthausen relates that those who dreamed that they were on their way home or that they were already there did not survive.

·

A possible explanation for the Prophet's *hadith*: "God loves the sneeze and detests the yawn." Sneezing expels demons and releases demonic ferments. There is liberation. In yawning there is absorption, a surrender to evil forces. That's why you put your hand over your mouth, to plug up the leak.

·

According to the Sabbath tract, there are three reasons why a Jewish woman might die in childbirth: for failing to observe the rules on menstruation, for neglecting to make challah (the sweet bread to offer to God), or for not lighting the Sabbath candles. But did the puerperal epidemics spare Jewish women who received the Sabbath with their candles burning? Saturn devours. Today there are Jewish women who don't give a damn about menstrual impurities, who bake cakes as offerings to non-exterminating faces, and who turn on the television set Friday nights without a thought for the Sabbath at the door. And they do not die in childbirth. Asepsis, cesarean section, safe maternity. Yoga exercises for a painless delivery. In the shadow of the future world, the rabbis look out sadly over the failure of their moral certainties and sigh over the unlit candles in rooms where an animated, talking piece of furniture crushes the corpse of the Sabbath.

.

Praesagium mortis ab odore. A mother asks the doctor what sign made him so certain that her baby girl was dead. "A faint odor of earth," he replied.

.

Why did Lenin win in 1918, and not the Russian Constituent Assembly? Because the Russian people wanted to suffer, at length, enormously, immensely, and Lenin was the promise of fear, hunger, pain, the unknown, the bearer of an abject but sufficiently tragic Messianism; and behind him loomed the horrible Stalin, the dark mold of a regime created to grieve and threaten Russia and the world. Neither Martov nor those poor constituents squashed by Lenin's fist could promise such unhappiness to a great people who refused to accept only minor suffering. Dostoevsky had no doubts: "I am sure that mankind will never renounce authentic suffering, that is, destruction and chaos."

.

If the world was created by Evil, it should be destroyed by Good.

·

Just as the blind wear dark glasses, the preternatural anus applied a tinted monocle to an eye that was already deprived of light.

·

The ideal instrument for a paralytic condemned to death is an electric wheelchair.

·

Do not urinate with excessive discretion: *Mingere cum bombis res est saluberrima lumbis*—Urinating loudly is very healthy for the kidneys, according to the teachings of the Salerno school. Proponents of Claudius' decree (which authorized such noises) should put out their own newspaper.

·

Art has been dead ever since artists stopped suffering from venereal disease.

·

If you gave that nag a scythe—Quevedo says about a broken-down animal—the other horses would think she was the Grim Reaper.

·

The Rig-Veda 112 consecrates all sodomy with the line: "The penis searches for the two hairy slits."

·

On deserted planets where there are no humans, light and darkness follow different rhythms. They are not pressed by the need to alternate Good and Evil, in the figures of Day and Night, within the narrow conduit of human hours.

The Silence of the Body

If, as their punitive destiny, only the worst specimens of human evil ended up on the anatomy table, we would be left with the hope that there was some essential morphological difference between their hearts and the hearts of the good, left closed and unexplored.

•

A free state, says Montesquieu, is one that is always agitated. He is contradicted by the Swiss republic and by England. Italy and perhaps the United States prove him right. Freedom without calm is preferable to its opposite, especially if you love calm. Without freedom, the stifled agitation produced by repression is much stronger or is vented in arbitrary acts of power that offer some release.

•

With the triumph of dentures, Edgar Allan Poe's tale "Berenice" loses its bite.

•

Every public bathroom with sit-down toilets should post this warning: "Sit here at your own risk." It would also be opportune in the home.

•

The surviving passengers of a plane lost in the Andes ate their dead companions for nourishment. Jumbo jet, maximum security, altitude of twelve thousand meters, from one hemisphere to the next in a few short hours; synthetic meals, television, movies on board—but in the end true man, natural man, turned into a cannibal by hunger, the nameless horror, the punishment of that absurd comfort. End of an illusion.

·

Le Rouge, the sorcerer, says the city witch doctor was often a failure at medicine, journalism, or literature and had to leave his province after many years there because of some scandal.

·

A man in gray, covered with scratches, is coming out of the woods, and to protect my female companion, I hold him off with a very long, thick walking stick. But the man follows us all the way home to our apartment, which has become a kind of asylum for half-crazed people, including my mother, who is in perfect health. The man (in reality a werewolf) tries to ingratiate himself and confesses his lust for me. With loathing I push him away. Thinking that I like one of the patients, a brutish type in a black plastic jacket, the man gets into a jealous argument with him. Concerned that the fight will end badly, with stab wounds, I leave the two alone to insult and punch each other and I go away, if only to be rid of the presence of at least one of them. A little while later, in comes the man in the jacket with a knife in his hand, soaked in blood; the other man is in the corridor, stretched out on the ground. I shout that a crime has been committed, but deep down I'm happy that it ended this way. I ask the concierge if there is any mail, and I worry how I will answer the investigators while I am about to begin a course at the university. The killer is sad: he is sitting on the floor of the landing surrounded by silent neighbors, and he says he is upset by what happened and does not understand why he did it. (But I know why, since I, silent interior instigator, wanted him to do it.)

·

The Silence of the Body

Borges considers the thirteenth-month bonus one of the moral outrages of Peronism. He is right. It is terrible to be paid for work that is not done, for time that has not been put in, for a month that does not exist. You could pay more for work actually done, but the invention of the thirteenth month is shameful. So is *severance pay* when employment is terminated; sometimes it is absurd, senseless. A man who has been *severed* is a dead man. "They have to pay my severance." It sounds bad. It smells like a crime. In fact, it is a moral crime. You should be *compensated*, not severed. If there is no reason for compensation, the money is corrupting: it corrupts you even if the only thing you have to give in exchange is retirement and idleness. In Rome, the *sportula* was less corrupting: it was compensation for running in the mud behind patrician biers, for flattery. The thirteenth-month bonus pays for nothing. It is hollow money, even if it is in circulation; it is the hole in hollow money.

·

According to Bichat, the *ultimum moriens* (the last thing to die, where the ultimateness of the *ultimum moriens*, the heart, is concentrated) is the black blood ventricle. *Ruit nox* (night falls).

·

In old people, after almost all the sensations of pleasure have been lost, taste is "the last thread from which the happiness of living is suspended" (Bichat). There is also a passage in Montaigne on the *sauces* that so preoccupy old age in the desert of desire.

·

Esquirol speaks a great truth: "Some individuals recover their sanity by leaving home and lose it again when they return."

The home fosters madness and nervous illnesses: *prison and dung heap*, in the words of the Buddhist. I love my home, but I am happy when I am far away. I do not see the bars, my reason is calm, my thoughts have freer rein, and my habits change. Those who have no home, who are born nomads, may never know mental illness.

.

An attack of hysteria is always preceded by epigastric aura with upward irradiations, a sense of discomfort, and pain in the stomach area, including nausea and cramps. Sometimes it is followed by vomiting, borborygmus, distension of the stomach, belching, hiccups, palpitations, and spasms of the larynx; then tetanus sets in, with the trunk bent sharply backward and the abdomen protruding. Chronic pain in the area of the left ovary is exacerbated during the fit (Solivetti, *Delle convulsioni isteriche*, 1884).

.

The political mental hospital is nothing new. "From Da Porto's testimony we know the Venetians used to lock up many madmen and the most outspoken critics of their government inside the Padua Castle" (Da Porto, *Lettere storiche dall'anno 1509 al 1528*).

.

According to Mesmer, an intestinal obstruction will arrest fluid energy until the obstruction is removed through magnetism. Mirrors reflect the fluid; sound transports it. The ancient occultists recognized the magic properties of mirrors and music.

.

Before the fifteenth century there were no insane asylums in the Venetian republic. The mad stayed home, but their relatives were hardly nurses: *Non custodiuntur in carceribus sed a suis coniunctis in suis hospiciis, ferreis vinculis alligati*—They are guarded not in jails but by relatives in their homes, bound in iron chains.

.

Rabbi Ben Hanna attributed the color of wine to the fermentation of the grape's ferruginous particles and their union through magnetism.

.

Paintings by Jan Steen: The chamber pot for urine always has a blue ribbon, a popular remedy against hysteria. An apron string was preferred, since it was usually greasy: the ribbon was burned, and the fumes, greasy and irritating, served to reanimate the woman stricken by *passio hysterica*. If the apron string had no effect, they tried an enema.

.

After the great plague of 1665, wigs fell out of fashion in London because of fear that the hair they were made with had fallen from plague victims.

.

If man had been given a bladder as big as an antelope's skin, maybe then he would not say: Why don't I have wings?

.

Semmelweis made his discoveries without sacrificing a single animal but solely through reflection and the examination of cadavers. Yet before the discoveries, many women died of infections received from his hands.

.

Man is a devil on skid row.

.

Man can no longer change or take another road; he can only come to a bad end.

.

Do you want to become a medical specialist? Then specialize, as did the most subtle Egyptians, in Unknown Illnesses.

.

At the climax or in the aftermath of a wild erotic act, sometimes a man's heart gives rise to the evangelical question Jesus asked his mother at Cana: "Woman, what have I to do with thee?"
    Baltasar Gracián says doctors form the march of death. They are "its most reliable ministers, unfailingly delivering death" ("La Suegra de la Vida").

.

Not everyone can create a painful syndrome (Leriche), just as not everyone can plunge into the crowd (Baudelaire). Lovely thoughts, which discover and preserve individuality in the most ordinary things (physical suffering, finding oneself in the midst of a crowd), and not only individuality but predestination.

.

Example of sadistic journalistic prose: "Of the ten stabs inflicted on Norma Mauro's body with inhuman ferocity, two struck her lower abdomen and breast. But the bikini the girl was wearing is not torn. A clear sign, maintain the investigators, that the man, probably a maniac, lowered the bottom and top parts of her bathing suit before striking.

The Silence of the Body

But Norma does not remember any of this. The only detail that stuck in her mind is that of a hand touching her body while the knife tore her flesh." (*Corriere della Sera*, July 22, 1973).

.

Thank you, Schopenhauer, for a thought that provides me with a broad justification: "It is really a very risky, nay, a fatal thing, to be sociable: because it means contact with natures, the great majority of which are bad morally, and dull or perverse, intellectually." More and more I too feel that contacting and seeing people wastefully robs the heart of its beats and the spirit of vital lymph. I know it is foolish to hope I will find someone in the crowd capable of giving to me or receiving from me anything good. "To have enough in oneself to dispense with the necessity of . . . company is a great piece of good fortune; because almost all our sufferings spring from having to do with other people; and that destroys the peace of mind, which comes next after health in the elements of happiness. Peace of mind is impossible without a considerable amount of solitude." (Look for these good maxims in *Counsels and Maxims*.)

.

Some forms of construction are far more damaging than any destruction.

.

Fornicate is from *fornix* (vault, arch; brothel), because in Rome the whores used to ply their trade under the vaults. Only he who fornicates in the open, under the heavenly vault, is a true fornicator.

.

"And how does that villainy increase and thrive? Through the religious sentiments of the democratic religion, which demands you speak of the rabble with respect; and if you call the rabble by its name, you are treated like an excommunicated heretic, as those who doubted Catholic dogma were in other times" (Vilfredo Pareto to Maffeo Pantaleoni, March 9, 1907).

•

A beautiful thin blond boy has abandoned the bodies of people he has killed on the terrace and in the rooms. The house is huge, with endless corridors, and seems almost like a castle. On the ground floor, maids are commenting on the events and policemen are warming themselves around the fire. The boy has disappeared. Fearing he has committed other horrendous crimes, they look everywhere for him. We go up to the second floor, and when the doors of the big armoire in the bedroom open, the child spills out, bound and bloodied but alive. We shout that we've found him, and the policemen come running. One of them picks him up in his arms. The boy cries, then he laughs; he's cold, and the good soldier consoles him, forgetting the things he has done.

•

Bestial is a very strong and vulgar word; *beast* is not.

•

Overpopulation and reincarnation. The subject raises once again the problem of the finite or infinite number of souls. Perhaps at the end of a cycle, all the souls that ever were are reincarnated with fantastic speed to drink deep one last time from the Ocean of Sorrow, whose waves grow even bigger and more frightening. Perhaps each demon strives to take possession of a human being, to frantically stimulate its generative powers in order to have more and more bodies avail-

The Silence of the Body

able. They battle to cause more suffering, more pain, well aware that this is their twilight, that the end of Time will leave them stunned senseless. Or perhaps God allows demons to dominate and entrance huge masses of men so that, with parsimonious grace, he may better choose his own among those wretched tormented souls. If the God of light is too distant or too powerless, Angra Mainyu becomes dominant, with a swelling in the number of souls that are prisoners of the flesh. Only a dark prince, a Sar Suma, could desire such a reckless increase in pain. But as the Epistle to the Romans says, Doesn't God take pity on us all by imprisoning us in evil (the deep meaning of *apistia*)?

.

A famous patriarch of the Eastern Church maintains that the dental nerve is a demon. I can feel it, but I am afraid that my dentist is a demon too (April 1974).

.

The bowels as the foundation, covered by a fluttering garment, pierced with seven holes and filled by the wind: man.

.

"I shall be like that tree, I shall die at the top" (Swift to Pastor Young, pointing to an elm tree whose upper branches were dead).

.

Attila the Hun got drunk at his wedding and died of a nosebleed during the night.

.

The newspapers are full of human sacrifice: they package crimes, accidents, and wars and make them acceptable to readers. In a certain sense the papers ritualize and organize these events (commentary with breakfast); afterward they wash the altar or the track and are ready to start over again, on the very same page, with new victims and new sacrificers. The death penalty has been abolished? But we are living one vast death penalty, handed down by groups and by nations. The nightly news is an execution update. There is much talk about *nuclear holocaust*: it is one of the language's most successful expressions, blending the ancient word and the new. The *caper*, the scapegoat, has disappeared: all the killing is meant to fill the void left in modern civilization by the animal that atoned for human sins! Haphazardly, pointlessly, but always *coldly*—the essence of sacrifice.

The powers-that-be claim to abhor human sacrifice and say that they cannot use the justice system to restrain all the assorted thugs and thereby sacrifice them in turn. Thus thugs end up in charge of sacrificing victims on *lay* pretexts, which at least protect the *tantum religio* from blame. The Manson *family* as a group of sacrificers adapted to contemporary life: they got around in a trailer and had a gas-burning stove and camping equipment. They took drugs, and at night they raised the sacrificial knife over the chosen ones.

In the Mass, the simulated sacrifice of the lamb is afraid to appear and cloaks itself in new words; outside the churches, fury and rivers of blood. The city becomes bloodier, its streets crowded with cars that maim, wheels that crush, and fumes that poison their victims.

The prophets of Israel placed all blood on God's hands; by making him the sole sacrificer, they relieved the city of the duty to slit its veins. But if God is not the sole sacrificer, then the city somehow feels the need to become the altar and valley of Hinnom, the hand that immolates. To grab our attention, to tie our hands, the law has to swiftly reinstate sacrifice. And they say they abolished animal sacrifice! They abolished only the ritual: they uninterruptedly, limitlessly, and needlessly exterminate animals. No, we have not replaced blood with paper and shadows. Paper, voices, shadows are there to reassure society, which fears there is not enough sacrifice. But there's plenty of sacrifice! With the expression *nuclear holocaust*, human society as a whole has adopted the idea of its own sacrificial consummation (not to obtain something but to atone for everything).

.

The sacred is frightening. But so is its absence, so is the desecrated world, void of rules and prohibitions. In freedom we cannot exist. We have to choose which fear is most consoling.

.

Why couldn't Lot's daughters have found someone else to get them pregnant? After the destruction of Sodom (where they would never have found husbands) there were still the neighboring cities. They could have avoided brutalizing an honest father with alcohol to use him for reproductive purposes. (Pascal praises this incident, because it is Scripture.) But there would be no *daughters of Lot* without incest; incest is what makes them become Scripture and, as Scripture, worthy of praise from the observant. Since the Righteous Man committed the sin in a state of drunkenness, he remained extraneous to his sin; as our laws would put it, alcohol was an aggravating circumstance.

.

A wisdom that passes, a Light that suffers: live with this secret.

.

Under the roofs, a huge room with many beds. I turn on the night-light to write, standing up at the table, and there is a woman in one of the beds who wants to sleep. "Ah, is it you?" (But I hardly know her.) I caress her fair hair, then a slightly cold kiss of mutual courtesy. Uncovering her, I find a cunt done up like a garden, with arabesques of hairs and painted flowers (yellow); a golden needle is sewing it up horizontally. After I kiss her, black paint remains on my lips. I go to a small mirror. My hands seem to be gloved in the paint. I have to cut the glove, while my mouth fills with disgusting black paint, which I yank out in thick lumps, yet it won't stop gurgling. Finally my mouth is free. I heave a sigh of relief, but I am afraid of the poison that has seeped in. (The second part is a syphilophobic dream.)

•

Alkaliubi advises the following: To preserve good eyesight, avoid excesses in coitus, crying, sleeping, staying up, bathing, and staring at small, white, or shiny objects; avoid onions, lentils, and beans (all the flatulent foods). To give the eyes luster and strength, eat a handful of unshelled, salted Mahalla lupine seeds every day.

•

Paracelsus says that the astral body, the procreator of incubi and succubi, secretes psychic sperm. (Lilith impregnates psychically.)

•

Flatulence from ingesting fava beans, according to the Pythagorians, is caused by the spirits of the legumes' dead inhabitants. Once they have entered the body, they torment the person who ate them: by day with gas, by night with nightmares. The nightmare is supposedly like an unexpelled wind that circulates internally, rattling the blinds that protect the sleeping soul.

•

The Silence of the Body

"They will dry their tears but burn the cities" (Dostoevsky, Notebooks for *The Possessed*). Anyone who dries tears with fire ends up with charred, empty sockets.

·

Water is the element opposite to Sloth. An enema proves it.

·

From Leopardi's poem "Incendio." While the flames devour us, the poet's warning tolls melancholically: "Nature wants to be enlightened by reason, not ignited."

·

It is soothing to think of the unknown and tremendous moments of human existence—spiritual creation, love, and death—repeating to us with their profound unknowability that everything comes *ex alto*, that the origin and the end, or the non-origin and the non-end, are not casual but inaccessible and distant.

·

I tell the gentleman to kiss the hand of the immobile old woman in the corridor three times, and then I will conjure up someone from whom Satan himself would flee. As soon as the gentleman lets me know that he has kissed her hand, I strike a saber on the floor three times with tremendous force, invoking the name of the Marquis, and the floor begins to shake and becomes soft, sticky, and as hot as boiling tar. Like chickens we roost on a piece of furniture and wait. Through the gaping floor rises the Marquis from his Charenton days, old, fat, enormous, bare-bellied, in a greasy, tattered jacket and shirt, his eyes evil and crazed, acting as if he wants to hurl himself at us. Satan, who was standing behind us, suddenly disappears, leaving a hole in the wall. I caress my father—he too is old and paunchy—to comfort him.

.

A caress arrives like the wind; it opens a shutter but does not enter if the window is closed.

.

Martin Luther, in *Table-Talk*, condemns suicide but absolves its victim as being in thrall to demonic power, and thus in a certain sense *murdered. Jehoshaphat:* God will judge him. "Nevertheless these things must not be taught to the people, so as not to offer Satan the opportunity to carry out massacres."

.

In the boundless ocean of human enslavement—to Fate, to Predestination, to the Cycle of Birth and Death, to the body, to the passions, to the Zeitgeist, to social order—political freedom is a mysterious gift, a flower blooming out of season. To lose it is to return to the normal human condition.

.

Edgar Allan Poe's "Mesmeric Revelation" speaks of a tuberculosis victim whose asthma attacks are relieved by applications of mustard to the nervous centers.

.

Master Pedro, the puppeteer in *Don Quixote*, is probably hiding a case of the French pox. Cervantes notes the disease only in Pedro's second appearance (II, 25): "He wore a green silk patch over his left eye and half his cheek, a sign that that side must have been diseased." Diseased, he is more picaresque.

·

In the Bolzano museum there is an Assumption into Heaven of Mary Magdalene amid Angels. A victory for democracy. Immediately after the Virgin, the lowly courtesan.

·

"An era so well informed about Energetics has lost the notion of the enormous forces hidden in an offering of a piece of bread" (Jünger, *Strahlungen*, February 1945).

·

Thérèse Raquin: the system of temperaments and its failure, the final victory of the purely fantastic. If they had been predictable fictional devices, Thérèse and Laurent would not have gone mad in such an extraordinary way, creating situations that might arouse the envy of a Poe. But beneath Zola's genetic code and physiological determinism lies a mythic code, and Zola often mistakes one for the other, with excellent results. What remains is not a monotonous physiology of temperament but the tragic profile of fatality.

·

To cure love sickness: *stercus amatae sub cervical positum—* the beloved's excrement placed under the pillow (Burton, "Cure of Love-Melancholy," *Anatomy of Melancholy*). But what if the lover is coprophilic?

·

Huysmans treated his cough with ice-cold showers; they helped. "Then I spend my time at the baths, exhibiting my shivering skeleton to the gaze of a fireman, who crushes my spinal column beneath the columns of icy water" (letter to

Zola, June 19, 1882). You can look it up in Veysset, *Huysmans et la médecine* (1930).

•

Had the industrial system not been forced to *improve itself*, it would have trembled its last on the threshold of this century; it could never have sustained such inhumanity and torture. But flying to its aid came the occult arms of Evil, social humanitarianism, literary philanthropy, unionism, Marxism, laborism, and even religion; redemption, progress, salvation. But you have made evil look nice, improved the vampire's breath, and put velvet gloves on ruthless claws, so the claws have kept on tearing. The industrial system stops being destructive and swallowing human lives in its furnaces only to destroy us with unanimous approval and to become the system of Universal Destruction. In some cases, industry is also a liberator, nourisher, and conserver of immaterial goods through monetary donations; it eliminates pain; it has itself worshipped as a benevolent God, as the only God. Now that the industrial system has convinced us to accept it, it can cast all of us into the fires of the abyss.

•

The beverages of poverty: tea in the Casual Ward and in the Workhouse, coffee in the mining villages of Zola's *Germinal*. Familiar drugs in the homes of the rich.

•

In the inn's courtyard there is a huge bearded gray pig—disemboweled. We cover our eyes, we run away. On our return everything is done: the pieces of the animal lie clean and in order, like the pipes of a disassembled organ.

•

The Silence of the Body

"The dead almost always look peaceful and serene, indeed liberated, as if the dust were happy to be free of the Spirit, and vice versa" (Hebbel, *Fünftes Tagebuch*, July 10, 1854).

.

Anyone who tolerates noise is already a corpse.

.

Society has begun to use neurosurgical wards to prevent crime. First there were infinite tortures, the supply of which will never end. Now they have been replaced by infinite operations. The unyielding ban on capital punishment foreshadows the extremism of monstrous therapies to treat the risk of excessive crime. They will try to turn murderers into chimeras, into empty, wandering shells, nervous blind men, amputees who only look whole, and ravaged, bent forms with half a brain. All for the sake of denying them the dignity of a conscious death in atonement for their crimes.

.

Beatrice Cenci, beheaded at the age of sixteen for patricide (she was not unjustified, according to contemporary accounts). Clearly she had to atone for her crime, but the Pope chose the horizontal guillotine, a pure barbarity in response to a complex deed. He may have placated the *Manes* of her father, Francesco, but he aroused the furor of Beatrice's. (With his compassionate paintbrush, Guido Reni partly righted this wrong.) Beatrice stands between guilt and innocence, in a highly precarious position, on an undefinable line, which makes justice painful and impossible to balance.

In our own times, Patrick, who was also sixteen, and an accomplice set fire to a school in Paris. They did not behead him. On the contrary, he immediately became a body with a hundred heads, the heads of the psychiatrists-psychologists-criminologists-social workers who flew to him with a single goal: to *rehabilitate him* into Society. But Patrick burned twenty-three children alive, made them vanish from the world: can his crime be absolved, forgotten? As a sixteenth-century judge, I might have punished Beatrice with poverty and Patrick with the galleys. As a twentieth-century judge, I would not know which side to take: poverty is an inapplicable sanction (Beatrice would immediately find a great job in television), and nonpunitive jails have taken the place of galleys, whose bitter water would have moistened the sores of the twenty-three who were burned alive. The guillotine exists, but no one at the age of sixteen is capable of understanding why he or she receives it. The only thing left would be to assess Beatrice one lira in damages, leaving it up to society to make Patrick into an acrobatic fire extinguisher (preferably of oil wells). Justice loses; but in compensation, cruelty and vengeance do not gain. Maybe the supreme punishment for Beatrice would be to take away Reni's portrait. If we still weep over her, it is thanks to this painting suffused with magic compassion.

•

Day (Helen-Pollux) and Night (Clytemnestra-Castor). Born from two different eggs, embodying the *duo principia* of Faustus of Miletus.

•

"Your purse or your life." With its purse, a kangaroo would be giving up its life.

•

The theatrical robots who represented Wagnerian characters began to vomit a yellowish substance with the violence of lava. The vomit dripped from the stage, flooding everything.

Marxism and Communist propaganda have infected the literati, making them believe that one who does not subscribe to the visions, ideas, and language of the left is not very intelligent and *not very alive*. The literati mistook the Communists for Impressionists who could not be rejected, without risking posterity's condemnation. "It's true, I don't like them, but they might become extremely valuable! What if they got into the Louvre someday? What if they went for millions at auctions?" And so they stuff their heads with venerated idiocies. If Impressionists, Cubists, and Abstractionists had remained outside the art markets and museums, the intelligentsia might better resist the blackmail of the cunning.

·

Vilfredo Pareto was the anti-Leopardi, the prophet of a humanity without illusions. Leopardi was torn between myth and reason; Pareto wished to eradicate every last remnant of human fable. He was a great unconscious destroyer of happiness, a bearded geometrist, admirable, and dangerous. He lashed out at the socialist illusion as the road to disaster, and time and events have proven him right. But when he attacked the ancient illusions, he scraped away life, extinguished the living soul, and joined forces with the socialism that destroys them.

·

A nice maxim from Napoleon: "However little you may eat, you still eat too much." Old age can be felt in the gullet; it enters through the gullet. But that ascetic warrior ate even his meager rations too quickly: eight minutes for lunch, fifteen for dinner. The result: an ulcerous stomach, chronic illness of the intestines and liver, and cancer due to digestive

disorders and neglect. Impossible to be worse off than Napoleon. The maxim is good, but the example needs correcting.

.

In Leopardi the enormous central theme is the destructive
truth, whose deadly rays kill our ability to tolerate life.
Thoughts, cantos, parables, letters, all his work addresses
this theme: his work is an uninterrupted spasm of pain, an
infinite weeping. Leopardi is the absolute anti-Marx, anti-
Hegel, anti-positivism, anti-progress. He writes for the sake
of the rare tokens, the few glimmers of the immutable atoms
of available happiness (either that or nothing, either the
blessed phantasms or desperation). He also glimpses the horror of the world unified under a single government: the
adorned uterus, the starry utopian canopy, the buttery Cana
of all the liberal, totalitarian Enlightenment men, the *ultima
Cumaei* of the Messiahs of matter. For Leopardi the unified
world would instead be the work of a degraded wisdom, a
final curse in the history of humankind: "Everywhere the
very names of nations and homelands will become extinct;
all mankind will gather . . . in a single nation and homeland
. . . and profess a universal love for their entire species; but
in truth humankind will scatter into as many populations as
there are men. Thus with neither a homeland to love nor
foreigners to hate, each man will hate all other men, loving
only himself out of the whole species." Leopardi did not fore-
see the fragmentation into groups, into sects, the massive
unification around idiotic utopias. Even the small nations are
rising: Biscay, Brittany, Wales, Catalonia, Corsica, Sardinia,
Croatia, each with its weapons, its armies of shadows, its
borders . . .

.

Done for. "Prosperity brings with it an elation that inferior
men can never resist," Balzac remarked. Populations consist

mainly of inferior men incapable of resisting this bliss. The destructive capacities and cravings of these former paupers of the West are amazing. And if one day Africa and Asia shed their impoverished masses, they will become mere fragments of uprooted nature. Prosperity is the flood, the plague of the Tombs of Lust.

.

In *Nana*, Zola says that tuberoses have a human smell when they decompose. Unfortunately, when man decomposes he does not smell like tuberoses.

.

The leg that you wash tonight could be amputated tomorrow. (But at least the surgeon will say, What a clean leg.)

.

The ant that climbed up the mountain of flesh and slid into its crevices sighed: "Clairvoyants speak of a spark, of an omnipotent intimate center, of a one-inch-tall inhabitant who is really a giant in disguise, and I walk across these rolling deserts, these forerunners of future rock, and I see nothing, I find nothing, nothing appears to me!" The ant's melancholy is justified, but the blindfolded clairvoyant in the depths is to be envied; he received tidings of joy, which his gesture sprinkles over the mountains of blind flesh like arcane benedictions.

.

The difference between a deep coma and imminent death is that sometimes it is possible to teach a comatose patient a certain alphabet (flickering the eyelids) that keeps some communication alive. But in other cases there are residues of consciousness that cannot be signaled: then you are in the icy grip of imminent death, held on the threshold of premature burial by the humiliated beating of the *ultimum moriens*, which can, however, be wrested from you for a transplant.

·

"What's better? To have Fun with Fungi or to have Idiocy with Ideology?" asked Aldous Huxley, who chose mushrooms (*Newsweek*, May 9, 1966). The rational choice is to flee mushrooms as ideology, and ideology as mushrooms. We'd be better off with no drugs.

·

The Spartiates prayed to the gods, "Give us the strength to tolerate injustice." They should have added, with the Helots in mind, "And to commit it."

·

Satire is a superhuman act, because it takes greatness and courage to figuratively trample on human dignity.

·

In a big, heavy Gospel I read a new Sermon on the Mount, in which all the Beatitudes signify—according to an interpretation in a footnote—that the only Beatitude is to die. "Blessed is he who receives a kidney stone" (that kills him) and other things of that sort. Suddenly a hand squeezes my balls ferociously, and while I struggle desperately to loosen his grip with my hands, a demon hollers insults and scorn into my ear, urging me, perhaps, to renounce him before he succeeds in hurting me even more.

·

With a little effort one can understand that even the hole in an outhouse is Shaar-ha-shamayim, *ianu coeli* (by the gate of heaven), but more crudely represented.

The Silence of the Body

•

Faces of blind Mongolian hordes will leap out of the elevator as soon as it reaches the ground and will light up in subway cars that have suddenly gone dark and stopped.

•

In Dijon, an Algerian who slit an old woman's throat to rob her adopted this defense: "I pointed the knife at her, but she started struggling and killed herself by rubbing her throat against the blade."

•

Embryotomy was a common practice in Rome to save the mother, and all midwives performed abortions. Roman law never considered homicide of the fetus.

•

They were closing all the doors, and the streets were quickly becoming deserted. It was day, but time stood still. It was said that a great flood was imminent, and the people barricaded themselves in their homes with enough provisions to hold out for a long time. I was especially shocked at the livid color of the light and the mute language of those closed doors, all in a row, which represented the whole city, concentrated in a single street. I went back in and ready hands immediately closed my door behind me. No one else could go out; perhaps no one else would ever go out.

•

As AIDS spreads in epidemic proportions, anorexia will decrease. Women will love themselves more, in order not to frighten men, whom contagion has turned into monks.

97

·

I struggled to climb an enormous stone staircase, feeling heavy and with a pain in my rectum caused by cancer. When I reached a dark curtain, which I opened, a great nave, or something between a closed nave and an open-air theater, appeared to me. In the background a Jewish or Masonic ceremony was taking place, with many symbols, mantles, and white cowls. "Jerusalem! Jerusalem!" I shouted from the uplifted curtain. Then, after a silence, again: "Jerusalem! Jerusalem!" I started to leave. Downstairs there was a flea market of dusty phonographs and records, and one of them carried my hoarse cry: "Jerusalem! Jerusalem!" The recording bore the full brunt of my unspeakable grief.

·

Certain American psychologists advise you to give babies fake excrement to play with to keep them from becoming coprophilic or coprophagous. But the opposite could happen: have they thought of that?

·

Nourished on the blood of a schizophrenic, a spider weaves crazy webs (Nicolas Bercel, "Araignées schizophrènes," *La Presse Médicale*, May 1957). The human civilization that is dominant today is a schizophrenic giant who methodically inoculates all living nature with his blood; and the spider Earth makes desperate and ever more fragile webs on which we set our iron feet, the feet of homicidal madmen.

·

Only woman knows how to love, says Marañon, because she knows how to disappear into the other. Well, certainly, disappearing into armoire-man may not be very pleasurable, but if no one disappeared into the other, we would all be visible.

.

"But didn't God make a mistake in putting the Jews in Russia, where they would suffer the pains of hell!" writes Isaac Babel. He doesn't see that it was no mistake at all.

.

"And should you love such a thing [anatomy], your stomach may still hold you back," said Leonardo da Vinci, but his love overcame his stomach. He seems to have been as indifferent to the death of men as he was to the fall of states, but not to the imprisonment of a bird. For him the birds sang the words of the Psalm: You have delivered us from the bird catcher's net. The final Flood, whose waves will cover every human horror, is his extreme message. His self-destructiveness can be seen in his semicryptic writings, the work of a fake left-hander, work abraded by erasures to annihilate thought. "It seemed as if he shook every time he started painting" (Lomazzo, *Trattato della pittura, scultura, ed architettura*).

Vasari's *mirabile e celeste* Leonardo was also the telluric speleologist of infinity, the man of flying dragons and terrifying Medusas, the prophet of the end of the world as essentially the *end of man* and his horrible organs of procreation. Thinking about Leonardo gives us both the joyous certainty that the Incarnation took place and the chill of its unknowability. He was the only Italian manifestation of Shiva, the ascetic and the destroyer. His red chalk self-portrait in Turin could be said to reveal the profound depression seen in the great thymopathic syndromes (Dalma, *Tendenze tanatiche in Leonardo*). But isn't it rather an inner exhaustion of the eye after such patient observation and inspection of the finite? Did he feel guilty for revealing too many things to a miserable mankind unworthy of knowing the secrets of life? The Turin drawing is an awesome *Deus Absconditus*. It is the smoke from two dying pyres: knowledge that has attained the most painful perfection and the nearness of the Platonic homecoming, whose price is the loss of being, because the soul longing to return home "desires its own destruction."

·

Putrification occurs very rapidly in a sewer, says Étienne Fournier's *Manuel de médecine légale*, and culminates in the saponification of the organic tissues. An observation applicable to the effects of the urban environment on morals (the *ethical fiber*) and on the social framework.

·

On July 6, 1802, Xavier Bichat fell while descending the stairs of the Hôtel Dieu. After fourteen days of agony, he died at the age of thirty from tubercular meningitis. He was a tireless Virgo (born September 11, 1771), and in his unlimited search for the functions of life, he divided every aspect of organic dissolution into a vast kaleidoscope. Research, dissection, and killing coincided in Bichat, a great thanatological worker and a frenzied lover.

·

In the *Recherches* (Part I, article 10) Bichat creates a physiological image of the terrors of death that bears a startling resemblance to the following verses from Leopardi's *Canto notturno*: "this supreme/fading of countenance,/and perishing from the earth, abandoning/every familiar, beloved companion." Bichat writes: "The idea of our supreme hour is painful only because it terminates our animal existence and suspends all the functions that connect us to our surroundings. It is the loss of these functions that sows fear and horror by our gravesides." Leopardi condenses the suspension of the functions in "fading of countenance," and the loss of all connections with our surroundings in the abandonment of every "companion," even a tree or a dog. Leopardi is romantically physiological just as Bichat is physiologically romantic. "Fear . . . by our gravesides" is a romantic figure.

.

Clothing that has been unbuttoned in correspondence to wounds is a sign of suicide (Cazzaniga-Cattabeni, *Compendio di medicina legale*). If the suicide were his own murderer, he would not undo his buttons.

.

Julian Gorkin's *Murder in Mexico*, on the assassination of Trotsky, contains the autopsy report, which in its nakedness attains a tragic beauty, considering the man killed and the circumstances. "The examination showed haemorrhage on the inner aspect of the lesion, that the orifice of the lesion was ¾ inch wide, 2¾ inches deep, and traversed the whole of the brain substance, with some loss of it . . . The direction followed by the weapon was from top to bottom, from the front to the back, and from right to left." The assassin was less ignoble in executing the crime than in plotting it; he attacked his victim from the front. This is how Trotsky escaped the second blow of the pickax. His left cerebral lobe weighed 1 lb. 6½ oz.; the right, the stricken part, 1 lb. 6 oz.: 2 lb. 12½ oz. in all. This is where the Bolshevik revolution was created.

While Trotsky's brain was in full activity when Death shattered its casing, Lenin's was three-quarters dead. The disease had begun several years earlier: at Smolny Lenin was already sclerotic, and maybe a premature sclerosis was the cause of his heavily repetitive, monotonous, and obsessive style, inherited by his repetitive, monotonous, obsessive, infantile, and sclerotic followers.

·

Better the soul suffer to see the body disemboweled and decomposed than it suffer from nonexistence.

·

In the gaseous phase of putrefaction every white man becomes black, and even a dwarf has his moment of gigantism.

·

Classic is the image of the impatient vulture spying on agony while resisting the urge to pounce. But even flies wait for the right moment to deposit their larvae, and in the dying man's room, sheltered and quiet, where the drama is consummated amid cleanliness and solicitude, and the vulture is mythic or exotic, how many scrawny vultures are spying on him?

·

The buzzing of the fly in Montaigne and Pascal. The good dipteron has no intention of killing your thoughts; it is attracted by your future corpse, or that something cadaveric which emanates from you.

·

Do wounds have individuality too? Two wounds can be very similar, but they will always diverge in some way. Their divergence lies not exclusively in the different structures of the receptacle but in something so ineffably and intimately individual that it modifies a mortal wound or the path of a bullet.

·

The Silence of the Body

Opinions. One person said that the smell issuing from Marie des Vallées's coffin was rosemary, another that it was spoiled cheese. The neutral people smelled nothing.

.

Pharmaceutical products for dogs and cats should first be tested on men kept in special cages.

.

"We are more sensitive to the Surgeon's incision than to ten slashes of the sword in the thick of battle" (Montaigne, "That the Taste of Good and Evil . . ."). The scalpel is awaited, but the sword arrives unexpectedly. We have stopped fighting but are forever waiting to enter the operating room.

.

Even in its superstitious forms—actually, because of them, since they are so full of mystery—religion preserves life. Spinoza, the most civilized of philosophers, brandishes the cudgel of a pure barbarian when he judges: *Quicquid in rerum Natura extra homines datur, id nostrae utilitatis ratio conservare non postulat; sed pro ejus vario usu conservare destruere vel quocumque modo ad nostrum usum adaptare nos docet.** He geometrizes the infernal principle of Genesis 9:2 ("The fear of you and the dread of you shall be upon every beast of the earth," the passage that makes Gnostics imagine Elohim as an evil Ialdabaoth). In this new guise, the old biblical principle triumphs, but henceforth shorn of admonitions and respect for the sacred.

Spinoza's *Ethics* IV, Chapter 26, reveals and teaches abstraction and insensitivity, yet we enjoy a tree and an animal

* "The consideration of its usefulness to us does not demand that we conserve everything that exists in nature outside mankind but teaches us, in proportion to its varying ways, to conserve it, to destroy it, or to adapt it to our purposes by every possible means."

as much as and even more than we do a man. Even when the *utilitatis ratio*—the utility principle—commands us to preserve, it is really working for destruction. This is proven by the failure of today's ecologists, who speak in the name of a conservative *utilitatis ratio* that has no authority in a world dominated by the destructive and that is unable to kindle a strong opposition. By doing whatever it pleases with Nature *extra homines*, mankind essentially brings about its own destruction. The *ratio utilitatis* exploits mankind too, otherwise it would not be completely *utilitatis*; this useful exploitation is Nemesis to taking what horror calls the final direction, after so much Hubris.

It was a tremendous error to identify God with human reason. Pascal speaks the truth: our *raison corrompue* corrupts all. (Leopardi translates *raison corrompue* as *arido vero*, the dry truth: the triumph of these two concepts is the means with which God chose to annihilate us.)

.

Noun construction in the Semitic languages: The main noun knows the dependent noun well enough to be modified by it. In the construction *bet-lechem*, "house of bread," bread becomes house, a content becomes container. More significantly, in Genesis 30:8, *naftulè-Elohim*—literally, "fights-of-God"—the center of the expression is "God" (the only possibility in biblical language). *Elohim* is an object that leaves its mark on the subject, *naftulim*, which would signify ordinary fights only if it had not been constructed in front of "God" (phonetic dependence is only the figure of a more profound dependency).

In his fine old tome on Spinoza, Giuseppe Rensi explains: "The torsion of the plate, the corrosion of the lamina, and the closing of the corollas are the knowledge these things have gained of the external fact that acted on them."

Here is the construction: The house, modified by the presence of bread, undergoes a morphological change. The house knows the bread well enough (like the fights that *know* God) to designate itself as house-of-bread, that which was transformed by bread into house of bread and not into house of something else. (This is a wonderful construction even when the privy is called "house of seat": the presence of the excremental seat modifies the room where it is placed.) The Semitic construction penetrates things more than our own genitive case does, because it expresses the deep cognitive relations between objects.

Rensi could have found more examples in Spinoza's Hebrew grammar, which presents various modes of cognition expressed by nouns. Even stronger than *naftulè-Elohim* is Genesis 2:4: *be-yom asot YHWH Elohim eretz ve-shamayim*, literally, "on the day of the Lord God making the earth and the heavens" (Vulgate: *in die quo fecit*, etc.). The cognitive relationship is lost in translation: the "making" (absolute state: *asah*, not a verb but a noun, according to Spinoza), becomes *asot* and assumes a different morphological connotation, modifying itself as if influenced to do so. In reality there is a virgin, inert *making* that God takes and transforms, *making* the heavens and the earth. Making is an object like "house," to which bread gives a face. That *making* is not just any *asah* but the "making" modified by the influence of the knowledge of God.

·

When the sunlight strikes its nose, the Statue opens up, and inside it a narrow pathway leads to the center of the earth. Diodorus and Melusetta descend by that path, finding themselves not in the center of the earth but in the midst of the 1793 Terror. (Perhaps the center of the earth experiences belatedly events that transpire on the surface.) Melusetta is accused of killing Marat, and her head is chopped off. Diodorus screams. They then pass by the Old Vampires' Home and various levels of hell, where they meet Hamlet and Hieronymous Bosch. An underground volcano will spew them out.

.

Like all rich doctors, Freud was a collectomaniac. His home in Berggasse was full of antique terracotta and bronze statuettes. The study where he had his patients lie down was swarming with these collector's items. They must have had a depressing effect.

.

The Josephinum in Vienna. Small, portable, homeopathic pharmacy from the first half of the nineteenth century; it is like a precious book, with six Lilliputian vials per row, all labeled. Maria Theresa's Penal Code of 1769 depicts various kinds of torture; the book is open to an illustration of a man tied to a ladder and pulled by ropes, receiving subcutaneous burns. (Detailed indications of the points to touch, like an acupuncture manual.) Hofmann's forensic treatise includes exquisite drawings of hanged men. Electroshock therapy session with Dr. Moritz Benedikt: whiteness of the naked leg of a female patient between the doctor's hands, the others lined up waiting in their overcoats. The *Tabakrauchklystier* was excellent: it helped impart to the lower bowels the joys of smoking. The scrotumless balls on the wax model of a flayed man create the strange impression of a double pendulum.

.

Armoire in a decrepit old hotel. Repulsive-attractive. It smells like aged yet still desirable female skin, *fascinatio dissolutionis*—the fascination of dissolution.

.

The Silence of the Body

Kafka calls the scrolls of the Torah "the same old headless dolls" but feels deeply the *mitzvah* of procreation. The Jew who does not procreate is himself a headless doll but the Jew who does not believe in God is even more of one.

•

Job and Sade. Sade is an aristocratic Enlightenment Job. Their common feature is lamenting the eternal *vice couronné*, the silence of a moral God. Together they recognize God's essential amorality, but this does not make the ancient believer deliver himself to evil. Sade is a henpecked Job: stricken by misfortune, he curses God. Perhaps Sade's condition, from Vincennes to the Bastille to Charenton (although he was a special, esteemed prisoner), is worse than Job's "among the dust and ashes."

•

Marvelous note by Thierry Maulnier in *Le Figaro* (January 22, 1977): "Our greatest adversaries since remotest time, both carnivores and herbivores, have ceased to threaten us since their disappearance."

•

I squatted and a piece of intestine came out of me; it kept coming out. My intestine piled up, lifting me so that I rose atop my intestine, which looked like a spiral column of gray marble. I rose higher than the houses, higher than the mountains, without ever separating from my intestine, which kept coming out. Finally I too was transformed into intestine, and that "I"-become-intestine was rocked by an internal explosion and came shooting down in the form of a star.

•

After making a long list of Pleasures and Pains, I discovered that the Pleasures were more numerous. We don't waste them—we live in them.

·

The only man who tied his name to the revolt against the machines of modern industry, the true, unfortunate bene-factor of humanity, is a man who never existed: Ned Ludd. Those good Luddites had to invent a leader to console them-selves in their solitude.

·

Implacable jealousy is typical of women who are mannish, or made so by menopause, rather than of very feminine women. Worrying about sexual domination belongs to the virile or-ganism and psychology (Marañon, *Climaterio de la Mujer y del Hombre*).

·

Marañon strikes a nice blow against the myth of youth: A man's sexual function begins to be truly mature only when he is thirty-five (the hero's age in Italo Svevo's novel *As a Man Grows Older*). His emotional life reaches its peak even later: "The true plenitude of man's heart, for love and for all kinds of delicate or passionate feeling, is not attained until he is between the ages of forty and fifty." Believing the op-posite, men superstitiously start loving at twenty or thirty, spreading disappointment and unhappiness with both hands.

·

Marañon again: The climacteric man's passion for young girls may disguise a homosexual inclination (the ambiguity or an-drogyny of pre- or early pubescent girls). Analogously, the climacteric man who is gripped by passion for a boy (according to Schopenhauer, homosexuality flares up at a mature age) could have a heterosexual inclination, because of little boys' rather feminine features: in reality, he would still be what he was, without any special attraction to the male sex. Plato explains it better: The mature man is more spiritual, more attracted to the Uranian Venus. He looks for the little girl with unformed features because she is more immaterial, more free from the earthly. His dissimulated homosexuality would be nothing more than a desire for love without flesh, without procreation, and for the raptures of conversation, whose aims are pedagogical (awful in men with confused ideas and insufficiently noble hearts), because man's immortal nostalgia and true homeland is Uranus. When man has fulfilled the procreation *mitzvah*, his eyesight is less clouded and his heart freer for love. The only thing he searches for in bodies is memory, the sign of the transcendent.

.

Desbarolles saw the scaffold in Lacenaire's hands (the head line on the palm split into two overlapping segments under Saturn). But the whole hand must emanate signs of active criminality or the deduction can be false and the sign simply indicate a mortal wound to the head. Moreover, one would have to be born in a country where the penal code dictates that all those condemned to death will have their heads cut off. Where the garrote or rope is the rule, will palms carry the sign of a strangled throat? When I called myself a "chirologist," I never saw hands with signs of death on the scaffold. After the abolition of the death penalty in Italy in 1947, all the signs that foretold it flew away from the hand, silently.

.

Hobbes is Spinoza's twin in his reflections on the *conatus sese preservandi*, the endeavor for self-preservation. Desire is what maintains and increases man's power over the world (it tends to increase insatiably). Pleasure is only a means; the true end is Power. (Sade's heroes have neither face nor heart; they are pure, objectified *conatus*.)

.

I discover strange old books in a small public square. At the entrance to an underground area, a delightful little Chinese woman who seems to be waiting for us takes Ar-Ar by the hand and leads her below, through a monotonous succession of communicating rooms; I follow the two women with growing apprehension over this mad foray. They stop in a vaulted room, very low, with walls of solid rock. There is a huge bed, and they make love. Afterward, the Chinese woman invites us to enter the Chinese Room. Another worrisome dash through those underground rooms, this time with the two of us together behind the Chinese woman, who guides us, smiling, to the Chinese Room, a nondescript bourgeois parlor full of Chinese kitsch, with jade knickknacks and lacquer furniture. The Chinese woman stays outside. I immediately think, What if she locks us in here? At that very instant I hear the door close and the key turn. I run to the other door, it opens onto solid earth: the Chinese Room was the end of the road. We make a tremendous mental effort to get out, and we succeed. Ah, it was a dream! We crack the dream like an egg, pop out into a large public square, and are now supposed to take the train in a subway station . . . No, no, rather than go down again we do not leave. We are happy to be out of there. But a very Chinese doubt comes to me: What if we are still locked inside the Chinese Room, dreaming that we got out?

.

If abortion is homicide, at least it has the extenuating circumstance of legitimate self-defense.

The Silence of the Body

•

What an image: Victor Hugo's republican hero, Gauvain, the former viscount who commands the troops of the Republic in Vendée, carrying a complete *nécessaire de toilette* with him through a merciless war, amid fires and ambushes. Man of war in a people's army, but always taking perfect, aristocratic care of his person, teeth, nails, etc. Feature of supreme nobility: "He had that effeminate air about him that is so formidable in battle." (Such a man was Bonaparte, the Androgyne.)

•

All physical knowledge bleeds. Behind how many busts of honored anatomists lie the bodies of condemned prisoners who were killed *pro studio di notomia*—for the study of anatomy? Behind how many great doctors do we find murderous experimentation on healthy, living men? Under Cosimo I, this was normal practice in Tuscany. Every now and then a condemned man was donated to Falloppio (*quam interficimus modo nostro et anatomizamus*—whom we kill in our way and anatomize), who killed him with soporifics and then explored him. The suspicion of similar practices hangs over the figure of Andreas Vesalius.

On January 15, 1545, Santa di Mariotto Turchi di Mugello, an infanticide sentenced to be beheaded, was *salvata per la notomia* and sent to the University of Pisa *ut de ea per doctores fieret notomia* (so that doctors might dissect her). Giulio Mancini of Siena, after being flogged and having his ears cut off for theft, was sent to Pisa *pro faciendo de eo notomia* (to be dissected) for sodomizing a boy. The boy, a more subservient version of Saba's Ernesto, was punished with fifty lashes at the post in the Mercato Vecchio.

But the anatomist Leonardo da Vinci would certainly never

have accepted the gifts that Falloppio used to accept. The impure and dangerous temple of the Cadaver can be penetrated with hands of light or hands of darkness. Might Falloppio have extracted from a poor infanticide whom he himself had killed the tubes to which his name is tied?

When the bezoar stone of Spain, a universal antidote, was brought to the King of France, he asked for the opinion of his celebrated master surgeon, Ambroise Paré. "Let's test the stone on a condemned man," said the surgeon. Quickly a cook who had been sentenced to be hanged for stealing two silver plates was brought before him. The cook was promised a royal pardon if the antidote worked. They gave him sublimate to drink and then some ground bezoar stone. His agony lasted for seven hours. Paré went to visit him in prison: the cook was pacing like an animal, his tongue hanging out, his eyes and face on fire, cold sweats, great retching, and blood spurting from his ears, nose, mouth, anus, and urethra. To *save him* Paré gave him oil, but too late; the cook died screaming that it would have been better if they had taken him to the gallows.

Paré himself relates this with perfect calm in his *Book of Poisons*. Once the cook is dead, he opens him up, checks his stomach, and finds it parched and dry, well cooked by the sublimate, as if a cautery had passed through it. The King orders the bezoar stone thrown into the fire. Behold superstition confounded and overcome by science: but that cook driven mad by pain lies in the balance of this victory. The Spanish stone was as useless as it was innocent.

.

Literally, *skeptikos* means "one-who-looks-around," who considers, weighs, and reflects. The opposite of skeptical is unbalanced, demented; even further opposite—the only person superior to the skeptic—is the inspired one, the *rishi*, the *navi*, the seer.

.

Zola, unpublished working notes for *The Dream*, quoted in Henri Guillemin's *Zola, légende et vérité*. Curious metamorphosis of Original Sin into Heredity, and of Grace into Environment. Servitude of the will, but the Environment can save. Zola provides life with no theological horizon, to avoid flattening it through the dogma of Heredity. But if God is not the Author of Heredity and Environment (of Sin and Grace), then they are merely two blind forces, with neither grace nor sin. (Laundryroom-Grace and Railroad-Grace save neither Gervaise nor Jacques Lantier: to save Angélique in *The Dream*, Environment is disguised as the Shadow of the Cathedral.)

.

Joubert says that we sense the aroma of tea more by taste than by smell. In fact, the palate is gently assailed by an aroma that the nose barely inhales. But in Joubert's time we had already almost lost our sense of smell and could only envy dogs. Sip your tea and do not despair. In the deep mental regions, where thought contemplates the Way and heaven curves its invisible dance around our painful efforts to penetrate it, the aroma of tea announces that heaven is near.

.

A failed writer can always become a successful judge on a revolutionary tribunal, happy with the power to kill innocent people with a huge, senseless apparatus.

.

At the moment when their enormous power in the Western nations could help avert the tremendous, mysterious threat of nuclear power plants, the labor unions have placed themselves at the monster's service with a rage, an intoxication with power, an arrogance, a stupidity, and an indifference to human frailty that forever covers them with shame.

.

Among the mega-machines of antiquity, Lewis Mumford includes the Egyptian pyramids, products of a mortifying, necrophiliac technology. All it took to make them work was a mummy.

.

Mankind will always choose a passionate hell over an inert heaven.

.

Theodor Adorno as an example of the intellect divorced from the heart. While his intelligence was lofty, its role was determined by this separation, and its stature reduced by the heart's absence. Too little connection between intelligence and heart in today's thinking world. Isolated intelligence, when it is not generating hells, can at best analyze them; it cannot raise a soothing barrier against pain. If the fire does not destroy us soon, we can predict centuries of endless analyses of hell, ever more refined and interesting. But we would be wasting our time to beg for a salve against the burns.

.

I never experienced any sort of pain, said Montesquieu, that could not be eased by an hour of reading. Now there's a true man of letters.

The Silence of the Body

An inner heteroadelphous, an invisible, fleshless twin brother, grows inside a baby girl and torments her. He, incomplete, with a terrible longing for a mother, releases himself through her senses, crying and wailing, terrified of being abandoned. The little girl, now an adolescent, finds peace only when the horrible little monster falls asleep. Sometimes he sleeps for weeks, but when he wakes, the rooms are filled and polluted with his harsh shrieking and his rumblings from a dark, demented well. Amazement and annoyance surround her; useless cures oppress her. Finally the girl tries to free herself from him through suicide, by throwing herself out the window. She is hurt but does not die. And there, on top of her wounded body, a sobbing little monster, a dripping fetus groaning with its own voice, looking for her nipple. The moment the rescue workers pick him up, he dies in their arms. The girl has a normal convalescence. Now she is free.

•

Erich Fromm is absolutely right to say that oral-genital embraces are not perversions, because perversion is characterized by a tendency to destroy, to suffocate life. (This is what Schopenhauer says about injustice, one will suffocating another.) Chamfort's maxim—Take and give pleasure without harming either yourself or others—is perfect for sexual relations. Perversion is harm done to others without their consent. (But even with their consent it is harmful, and suffocating the life or the will of others always harms the suffocator.)

•

Reciprocal gratitude is the sign of the success and the beneficial effect of a sexual act. But do not probe the sincerity of this gratitude too deeply. Stop at the surface of the smile and the words.

·

Anyone who does not speak or smile after lovemaking degrades Eros.

·

The symptoms of shyness, described by Montesquieu in the *Reflections*, resemble the turbulence of the lover's jealousy in Sappho's ode.

·

During cholera's visit to Paris, when rumors of poisoning led to massacres, Guizot said, "Civilization sleeps atop an immense mine of barbarity."

·

In a thirteenth-century miniature illustrating the *Cyrurgia* by the Dominican priest Theodoric of Freiburg (University of Leiden library), touching the rectum looks like a great kindness.

·

Certain prophetic almanacs were crossed with a recent philosophy, and an errant reading of Chaos with profane ideas of Geometry: the result was called the *French Revolution*.

·

In the space that separates the Buddha from Émile Littré, the French lexicographer, there may be a point where I can situate myself. The problem of salvation (of true wisdom) is *emptying oneself*, and all I do is follow my libertine curiosities, fill myself, devour the past, and chase ghosts through the corridors of Time. But the only true wisdom presupposes mental *kenosis*, emptying. The rest is Desire, the search for distractions. God can come only into an empty heart concentrated on him, and not into a heart filled with Dictionaries. Dictionaries are Sin at the door, ready to hurl themselves at you. By writing *learned* books, I in my turn will fill others, who will look to me for distraction, thinking that they are looking to me for knowledge. But incomprehensible human history, with its enigmas and abysses, gives us a sign and points to something beyond the barrier. The bloodied victims of spiritual and physical battles implore us to avenge them through the gesture of reflection, to do them justice through thought, and to give their senseless burning in life a sense, without which their shadows howl. Thus I try to justify an overwhelming pleasure. Have pity on me. Buddha, an adiaphorist, untangles the indecipherable; Littré, the sublime victim of prostatitis, confined to his armchair, compiles words in an enormous list of meanings; me, I'm a piece of seaweed, tossed now this way, now that.

.

Jünger says that even in Medicine, Tactics are variable and Strategy unchangeable. "The moving hand treats, the steady hand heals" (*Strahlungen*). This sounds like a Taoist maxim.

.

For Spinoza, Eden still exists, man never left it. Eden is the world, which we lack the courage to call Gan Eden. Such a thought redeems the world but deeply offends human suffering.

.

Poor Montesquieu! He said that the air in France compensated for everything; he only hoped that it would never be polluted. In 1720 the plague passed through, but it was not carried by polluted air. Today, the air that compensated Montesquieu is polluted, and the water has become undrinkable almost everywhere because of chlorine, chromium, and radioactivity. An honest man can no longer express such a simple thought in any part of the world.

•

I love Leopardi despite his indecent consumption of coffee and sugar, while Marat's excess in consuming coffee and sugar makes me hate him more. In the first case, they are poor sustenance for a sublime being; in the second, explosives that excite a rancorous, evil, tragic demagogue.

•

The killer who strikes you has a cruel face—the face of dark Vishnu. But where is his bright face in that moment? Right on the nape of his neck: a clear, smiling face, full of enigmatic grace, gazes out from behind. But you do not see it, and so you die with terror in your eyes. If we could see it, no killer would be frightening: we would realize that he is an illusion, a game, an averted face. Mary Kelly would smile at Jack the Ripper, Sharon Tate at Susan Atkins, and his hundred victims at Dr. Petiot from the peephole of his gas chamber on rue Lesueur. The more terrifying the killer, the brighter and more reassuring the face you cannot see.

•

"Sir, forgive me, I did not do it deliberately" (Marie Antoinette, on the scaffold, to her executioner, for having stepped on his foot by accident). Courtesy and Guillotine: these are memorable encounters! Apologies to a foot are a queen's last exquisite sign of superiority.

.

You can become wise by accumulating distant ignorances. Ethnology.

.

Bleeding the ear increases male sexual potency (Scythians, Turks, and Buccaneers). A ring in the earlobe as the mark of a strong man. Today, of a slightly eunuchoid anarchism.

.

To avoid overstating your opposition to modern revolutions, think of the bound feet of the women in China before the revolution of Sun Yat-sen.

.

At eight o'clock in the morning the view of Siena from Santa Maria dei Servi is a dream of Good Government: clear sky, sunlight, the fragment of a slanted wall that sharpens the view of the near distance. This vision of human creation is intensely moving when you realize that in this world and time it is unique. Siena in the morning, dry harbor of rested and active nerves, taut as a ship at Lepanto or a trireme at Salamis.

.

The urban morphology of Siena makes it more subtly oppressive than a chaotic, pulsating industrial city. You are inside the Labyrinth, a soft, implacable labyrinth. Streets turn into other streets. You pivot on invisible hinges, always returning to the same point; you begin the same walk again, past beautiful doorways leading to sealed entries. There are no trees, and there are walls everywhere; you fear you will never get out. Perfect city for religion: it used to be easy to get out of the Sienese labyrinth by gazing at the sky and thinking about it, concentrating on the figures of its inhabitants. Now that the heavenly way has been lost, you are a prisoner in Siena.

.

An example of perdition in the infinity of inanity: The newspaper reports that, in order to manufacture a hormone (somatostatin) in the laboratory, a researcher "obtained it with great difficulty from the pituitary glands of sheep. The experiment yielded a tiny amount: from millions of sheep pituitary glands supplied by butchers, he obtained one milligram of hormone." On one side of the scale, millions of slaughtered sheep; on the other, the Nobel Prize milligram. By today's economy, the milligram weighs more. But come, look at your reflection in that milligram of hormone: is there any reason to bestow a prize on the human face? And what of all the whales massacred to make Victorian corsets? Both fashion and science will always lead to shame.

.

Giuseppe Parini's "The Smallpox Vaccine," dedicated to Dr. Gianmaria Bicetti, is a masterpiece of Enlightenment poetry. It breathes a messianic air: a world without smallpox could have been a wonderful dream. But little by little the defeated diseases have vaccinated us against the dream of overcoming them.

.

In a study of Odilon Redon, Émile Bernard calls him a great lover of Bach and Beethoven. Redon writes in the margin that he did not love or understand Bach. Bernard also singles out Pascal and Poe. Redon denies this. For him Poe is too cerebral to arouse representations of living forms. I share his feeling: I could not even shake a puppet show out of Poe; he has no figurative substance, and leads you through a labyrinth of abstractions.

.

Since all of Svevo's *Confessions of Zeno* is the analytic confession of a sick man, its conclusive eschatology culminates in a universal healing: after the bomb's explosion, the earth will be liberated "from parasites and diseases."

.

Without a moral remedy, says Constantin Hering, medicines are useless (*Homeopathic Domestic Physician*). They are not only useless but harmful. And the great hunger of moral drugs will wander the earth, swelling more and more, insatiable . . .

.

Goethe says that medicine must absorb a physician's total being, because his object is the total human organism.

.

Martinetti on Kant's two infinities: "But if the moral law in us is a true absolute reality, if the moral order is the essential foundation of all reality, then what do the myriad stars in the sky matter?" This provides a key for understanding the prophets, those ultra-Kantians obsessed with the absolute reality of moral law, who for its sake would demolish the sky and stars.

.

Rereading "Silbo de afirmación en la aldea" by Miguel Hernández: the music of sorrow. A voracious and prolix poem (it goes on forever), it violently affirms the superiority of life in the fields—the true life—over urban Thanatos (the city as

121

a pure expression of death), with its spires and towering antennas of lyric dissolution. Hernández was the last poet who could bring true tears to the eyes of an intelligent heart. He was a poet with a rifle strapped to his shoulder, who fired only at death. His lament "What are you doing here, things of God?" (and he names the donkey, apple, cloud, stones, and roses) is one of the most religious in our time of singularly shattered and desperate religion. The city is outside God, hence its incurable ailment: the swift massacre of innocent, living realities. And today even the 1934 *aldea* (village) wears the leperous face of a city . . .

•

From the balcony on via B. we saw a big spaceship fly by, like the ones in *Star Wars*, a Soviet satellite loaded with plutonium that came down slowly, to disintegrate on impact, and there was great fear among us small, poor, ordinary people. The bomb fell over there, in the sea (from the rooftops of Turin you could see the sea). I raised loud curses at Hubris, and instantly my mouth was filled with radioactive salt, while the deadly cloud moved toward us from the sea. I took shelter inside an elevator, which turned out to be a rickety country outhouse, where a cat stuffed with straw poked its head out of the crack-riddled toilet. In the midst of all this my father maintained the enviable calm of a true Buddha.

•

In Poe's "Descent into the Maelström," there is rare beauty in the moment when the seaman is ashamed of having been afraid to die "in view of so wonderful a manifestation of God's power."

•

Catherine Eddowes's kidney, sent to Mr. Lusk by Jack the Ripper in his letter "from hell," was identified as authentic by Dr. Openshaw of London Hospital: it was permeated with gin and infected with a form of nephritis.

.

Zola the naturalist denies moral responsibility; Zola the Dreyfusard is forced to defend it (as was Spinoza, after the massacre of the De Wytts). Theoretically we can accept moral irresponsibility, but if we try to lead lives consistent with this principle we immediately gasp for air.

.

We drew cards, requesting the identity of Jack the Ripper. Was he the Duke of Clarence, Montague Druitt, Virginia Woolf's cousin, Oscar Wilde's friend, or an Unknown? The cards indicated the Duke of Clarence. One point in favor of Stowell's thesis. Infected in India in 1879, Clarence could already have been suffering from tertiary syphilis by 1888: there is a short but perhaps sufficient amount of time between the infection and the crimes in the East End. If this is the story, the knife that cut Mary Kelly to pieces in Miller's Court was introduced into the blood of one of the Queen's nephews ten years earlier by an Indian boy. Like the spread of the old pandemics, an invisible *rattus rattus* from Bombay arrives at the Thames, not in stowage, but in a luxury cabin. Jack is another plague of London, and he establishes his speedy, minuscule pandemia of fear in literature and in myth.

.

If we deprive loving feelings of the morbidity that lubricates them, we will become not *healthy* but sterile, atrophic, buffeted by the arid wind of cruelty.

.

We could have digested this huge change and upheaval of life, habits, environment, and mental customs if it had occurred over the course of a thousand years, a little longer than the period between the founding of Rome and the reign of Constantine: but in less than a hundred years! And in only fifty years, how many severed roots! And in the last thirty, a force of such terrifying brutality! And the ten years just past only further increased the imbalance! And last year! And next year could be worse than the last fifty put together! All we can do is lose our minds, as Forbes-Winslow predicted: indeed, we are out of our minds. Those of us who reason know we are speaking to an audience of demented people or candidates aspiring to dementia. The Europeans are an insane people. (It pains me to say "people": the unifying element is our common insanity; before going so mundanely crazy, we were intelligently dissimilar nations.) The African and Asian peoples are going mad even more quickly; they've never received so many whippings. America is a bedlam without walls. Russia is a deadly Medusa. The worst madness lies not so much in little acts of indecent insanity as in the refrains that lament insufficient speed, *wasted* time, *unavoidable* delays, and the risk of a *slowdown*. All plunge us into the fraud of this madness, to the bottom of the well, black with screeching fallen monkeys, where the tragic *Narrenschiff* spins like a top.

.

Pascal's thoughts on St. Theresa are enlightening (but the blade of his light often slices away the pressing truth): "What pleases God is the deep humility in her revelations; what pleases men are her visions." Humanly, in fact, the only things I love about St. Theresa are her visions; her humility irritates me, for it dilutes the visions. But why should God hate the visions, which belong entirely to him, and prefer the shadow of a mechanical humility?

.

The Silence of the Body

Woman had her safe, dull happiness: in completely aban-
doning her improbable existence to man's attempts to construct his and in becoming his material. Now that she
struggles to construct her own life, by herself, and fishes in
the great seas of man's unhappiness, she has turned into a
man full of holes, who immediately sinks.

·

We are ignorant of the world's hunger for love. There is
probably less love than you might think. Every day presents
us with occasions to appease this hunger, but we are unwilling
to break our fast, or we realize that we were never really
hungry.

·

Fuchs calls the *Ecstasy of St. Theresa* in Santa Maria della
Vittoria in Rome "one of the most immoral erotic works in
European art," an unfounded hyperbole. Quite simply, Bernini's sculpture applies the unapplied affections of Theresa
of Avila to the wrong object. Baudelaire knew that her affections had not really been unapplied; Bernini pretended he
was applying them to a mystical object but delivered them to
a "scorpion of the world's pleasure," with an Eros-cherub
giggling at her enthrallment. His work is a Baroque without
Spain and without Theresa, with the scent of the Pope around
the corner; it is far from her true cherubic ecstasy within
the walls of the Encarnación in Avila. The episode of her
transverberation was like slipping in a greasy kitchen and
breaking a foot, closing up a farmer's market at sunset, falling
out of bed while dreaming, exchanging greetings between two
windows where laundry is hung to dry. Nothing more *natural*
for a Theresa than to be transverberated as she thinks, writes,
or prays in her convent. If the Encarnación (at least Theresa's
section of it) were not a museum today, we would feel her

ecstasies entering us like the ordinary sounds of women, chickens, or footsteps in a country home. Her face reflected her diseased stomach and constant nervous tension, but it was wide, not gaunt or sickly. Theresa bore no resemblance to Bernini's languid woman. The statuary group is immoral not because it is erotic but because it is false, because it is a spiritual forgery. If the title were changed to *Sister of Loudon* or simply *Ecstasy*—the generic ecstasy of a morbid nun—it would shed its immorality.

.

Any speech on love that is not designed for a small, elegant society is wasted or in vain. If too many people are addressed, one doesn't know what to talk about. Today, in order to talk about love *to the masses*, the erotographer takes his bearings from the gestures of his audience and from the steam emanating from their crotches, convinced that he is talking about normal behavior and easily recognizable signs. But a common understanding of this seemingly elementary universal language would require a universal pornological education, a conversion *en masse* to the pubic and anal areas, which view all life in terms of excitation and orgasm.

.

Almost everyone finds Sade incomprehensible, and perhaps he always will be. In the meantime, however, the letters to pornographic magazines struggle to establish a code (if you're that big you'd better find yourself a hairy girlfriend; tear off your solitary disguise: it hides a frenetic seeker of ass; your sister should masturbate you; do not fear diving into menstrual blood). Statistical orgasms—the responses of thirteen thousand people to a survey conducted by two female doctors —aspire to become catechisms, travel guides, or entries in an almanac, but they leave the impression of penetrating deeper and deeper into a no-man's-land, with trampled fences, scorched by bombardment, stretching into infinity. Among the corpses of a silenced trench lie the remains of the statue of Aphrodite, covered with mud and blood. The march of reason unenlightened by the heart provokes the same effects everywhere, in every walk of life.

·

The prohibition against taking one's daughter as a lover is compensated for by permission to take one's lover, or wife, as a daughter. The converse of incest is *nomos* (custom, rule), which also has a certain morbidity.

·

According to La Rochefoucauld, jealousy causes gangrene, rabies, and the plague. And indeed, such epidemics have stopped since we learned to be more tolerant.

·

It is unfair to deny public men, statesmen, the right to a few private pleasures, because the public welfare depends in part on these pleasures. Kamandaki's treatise counts only four pleasures: hunting, gambling, women, and drunkenness. He wants the prince to be an exception. What attracts men to power today? In the West, vice has been greatly weakened, but the pleasures for the weak have multiplied. The greatest danger is the steady attraction that money exerts on public men. Money is not a pleasure but a disgusting disease. Their finances should be harshly inspected; if they are greedy, they should be driven out, thrown in prison, or sent to the gallows.

Tito of Yugoslavia always went hunting, but his attention to the state never wavered. Anwar Sadat found his greatest pleasure in watching Westerns, but this idiocy did not prevent him from managing the affairs of state. Many Italian ministers and legislators have a passion for soccer: it gives them some release from their degradation but aggravates it too—they need lovers! In classic fashion, Kissinger was partial to women: without this unwinding, this secret rudder, this holing up in a room every so often with someone who would finally make him waste an hour, his diplomatic intelligence would have become purely aerostatic, a flying ship battered by the winds.

But Gambling is disastrous, because it can make a person rob from the state, and drunkenness is disgraceful. Sometimes, however, a man needs a solitary session with a good bottle to collect his senses and make decisions that are difficult when his powers of inhibition are intact. Moderate doses of psychedelic drugs can be useful and can illuminate ideas: but it takes an intelligent statesman to make controlled use of them. A leader or minister should never be reproached for women (or boys), as long as he enjoys them within limits that are not modeled on Tiberius or Nero. Who could reproach Juan Negrín for spending a night with a whore from the Calle de Atocha shortly before the fall of Madrid? He would have spent that night either making unnecessary mistakes or serving no useful purpose to the state, since the game had already been lost. In the bed of a woman he has picked up on the street, the leader of a dying republic seeks only to hold off his imminent nervous collapse. The public man experiences dreadful tensions that surge in the midst of the crowd, in meetings, in constant travel, in assemblies; anything he can do to release them in private soothes the public welfare. Without private pleasures, the man who governs or legislates loses his human dimension, especially today. He is definitely a man of Artha. Kama must not prevail—beware if he takes the upper hand—but not even Dharma can free public man from the duties of Artha.

The Silence of the Body

In a lover's tryst, five times is really too many. James Boswell tells us this about himself, and discusses it; Louise says that for a woman twice is fine. Male hubris, insufficiently restrained by his Scottish origins. Her "twice" confirms the measure given by Tiresias: pleasure has nineteen parts, nine for the man, ten for the woman; since she has *one more*, she doesn't need repetition. But why in the world would a man need forty-five in a single tryst? Today, Western man begins to become ill at eighteen. True pleasure consists in seizing that nine in a single shot. And making it worth ninety-nine.

•

Lesbian love as humanity and freshness. Zola creates Satin (the "divine Satin," says Huysmans) to humanize Nana, when she is about to lose her human face, caught in the monstrous myth-producing delirium of her author. When Nana's mythological deformity makes contact with Satin and her "virgin blue eyes" (the color blue and virginity: Marian religion, water on the hot iron), it leaps backward, toward the Goutte d'Or district, her most human time, her lost *normalcy*.

•

Most women are bereft of the erotic sign, of that ineffable force that prepares them to attract love (and *to save it*, said the Alexandrine sectarians during the Gnostic era) and to transform it into disease and grandeur: cold, dark wombs, in which life is monotonously transmitted. The erotic sign surrounds the body with an aura, visible only to the well-trained eye or when revealed by *grace*. A woman is born with this sign, which is why some little girls can arouse true passion in perfectly normal men. She also dies with it, because old age disguises but does not erase the sign, and it still glows on hands that tremble and grow cold. Perhaps this sign condemns one to rebirth, but the old woman who has known how to love sees rebirth as a return to pleasure.

.

The most beautiful gesture of alienation from, and indifference to, the Christian world, time, the revelation, feelings, and Christian rites: an Eastern rabbi who, on Christmas Day (when it is forbidden to read the Torah), cuts toilet paper for the whole year. (Kafka tells this story.)

.

A woman is found asleep on a Monday morning, all curled up in a public trash can. She has lost her memory: she can remember only the pieces of trash with which she has lived, familiarly, since Saturday night. She remembers them affectionately, enumerating and describing them: a charming plastic syringe, two or three well-soaked tampons, potato skins as light as balloons, pictures of a little boy from fifty years ago, others of a man who is about sixty years old, one of a thirtyish man smiling with his wife in front of the Tower of Pisa, gray socks with holes in them, needles, a bra, pieces of glass, dead flies, two live worms of a pretty pink color, a wilted orchid, a pair of thin and still good gloves, overcooked pasta, chicken bones, a bag of vomit, melted strawberry ice cream, globs of mucus, an illustrated magazine, a number of clippings from hard-core pornographic magazines, a toothpaste tube with some paste still inside, cotton and gauze with dried blood, a pair of scissors, a nail file, a mechanical clown with the spring coming out of its stomach, a sheet of lined paper with a composition for school, lettuce leaves seasoned with too much vinegar, an empty bottle of vinegar, some shells, an empty matchbox, thirty-seven cigarette butts, a baby tooth, a pencil sharpener, a burnt-out light bulb, a drawing that didn't come out right, leftover fish, a crooked nail, an affectionate message, a full bottle of tonic, two rubber condoms, one used, one clean, a spot of cream, many buttons and pieces of colored cloth, four apple cores, a typewritten sheet of paper, an I.D. card, a teaspoon, and a penny. She feels as if they were her children, to nurture and protect. "I want to return to them, my life is there."

.

A flasher who has sneaked inside the Fun House at an amusement park takes the place of a skeleton gnashing its teeth. The cars of the little train arrive full of schoolgirls and he is suddenly illuminated by a red light: he is a laughing chimeric ghost with his genitals exposed and excited, an extraordinary, macabre Priapus. The girls laugh, scream, and cry. Everything stops. The flasher has disappeared: but from the skeleton hangs his spent, flaccid penis.

.

Jesus sees himself as the Resurrection from the dead, so he finds it absurd that some people, rather than follow him, waste time arranging funerals for their fathers. He commits Hubris. To avoid it, Antigone lets herself be buried alive; Hubris will strike back at the King twice. Defying Hubris is grave. Jesus defies it many times; thus whoever does not feel like sinning against divine laws cannot follow him. A tremendous choice remains, which few people have understood. Uprooted from all religion, we share the miserable thought that "burying the father" is a waste of time, a useless, ignoble waste. And we do it hastily, reducing the rituals and farewells to a minimum, so that everything is over *by ten o'clock*. And when everything is over, we have no one to follow, no Resurrection made flesh awaits us in our father's deserted house or at the street corner. We no longer speak with our dead father; we consider him completely dead, a diabolical absurdity. Finding his papers, we say "the dead man's papers"; if we take his old umbrella for ourselves, it becomes "the dead man's umbrella." We give him a minimum amount of time, negotiated in the fever of the hours, and pay the undertakers to do everything well, and with haste. Such stinginess would *bury the father*, a father truly believed to be dead! Perhaps a quick burial is no burial at all, and we commit Hubris, stupid, vulgar Hubris, without the grandeur of Jesus' defiance.

.

In ancient Mexico syphilitic *bubas* were at the origin of the World and the Sun, and syphilis was a cosmogonic disease. (Bubas were distinguished according to degrees and shapes —*Karqhia-xilim*, pointed gourds that grow, *Tzuputzak-xilim*, big gourds that grow, *Ahauh-xilim*, gourds of the nobles: the disease was a sign of aristocracy and shunned common people.) Similarly, Lucian podagra is born with the Sun and the Dawn. It is an epiphany: "And in that time the power of Podagra appeared." (But what if Lucian's omnipotent solar podagra was really *bubas* or *xilim*?) Fracastoro restored the myth of the disease's solar origin in an age of skepticism and science: the shepherd Syphilis is struck by Phoebus. If we free ourselves from the myth of Eden and the idea of the Fall, it is easier to accept the formidable connection between human disease and the origin of life.

.

"The *Bubas* appeared to be an exclusive attribute of wisdom, of science, and by extension of divinity, forming the basis of the indigenous faith, the foundation of its mysteries, or its sciences, and of its primitive civilization" (Don Mariano Padilla, *Ensayo historico sobre el origen de la Enfermedad Venérea o de las Bubas*, 1861). "And God saw that it was good."

.

A passage from the Aitareya Upanishad explains sodomy as the sexual form of the death instinct: "Death became the Descending Way, and entered the excretory organ." At its opening, the scythe-wielding, masquerading Old Woman casts the hook of Phoenicia. There is a close relationship between sodomy and coprophagy. At the bottom of everything is Atman striving to grasp Nourishment, and the Upanishad says that he can do so only through Excretion. All loves are ravenously hungry, but here there is a necrophilic hunger attached to the Descending Way by a *plaisir de descendre*, to degrade oneself totally, completely, almost a wish to decompose in a symbolic act (the poem "Ces passions qu'eux seuls"; obscene verses from Verlaine's *Hombres*: "Un peu de merde et de fromage"; Bressac's self-exaltation in Sade's *Justine*; Sade as both a perfect sodomite and a coprophage of the opposite sex). All this aside, popping out of the descending canals is undisguised Death: Here I am, ready for the final hunger, Crime, and Destruction. The biblical God, the living God and God *of the Living*, is rightly the enemy and destroyer of Sodom, *bet-hamavet*, necrophilia nesting in inhabited stones on the shores of a Dead Sea and not of a city of the living.

.

Descartes says that when love is neither sad nor too strong it is good for the health—the heart beats well, the chest feels a sweet warmth, and "meat is quickly digested in the stomach"—while hatred makes you vomit (*Les Passions de l'âme*). The indigestibility of meat is implicitly recognized if the stomach can only digest it when happily in love. *Omnia vincit amor*.

·

The true meaning of the Greek *ta aidoia* is "things that inspire reverence," "reverential fear" (since they are powers, the close contagion of the invisible). André Chénier is right to say that translating it as "shameful parts" is incorrect (*Notes philologiques*). The Greek word expresses respect that dares not approach, not ugliness to be concealed.

·

To feel Desire breaking away from the flesh is like watching the body break away from the soul to disappear.

·

We are fighting over scraps. In the poem "When They Are Roused," Cavafy says we should fight to preserve our erotic visions, capturing them the moment they come alive, with the melancholy knowledge that few will remain. Poetry as a small private museum of tiny collages and cutouts. Perhaps this is how we defend ourselves from the enormous, from the visible power of man that pulverizes us.

·

The aging man thinks he still has plenty of erotic energy to expend; the deceptive signals he receives are from an irritated prostate that has begun to tire.

·

The rooms fill with shreds of burnt skin that have fallen off: the love that disintegrates day after day, informing us that soon the only epidermis against raging solitude will be memory. But how many couples still have clean, spotless floors, having never had a living love from which something dead might one day fall!

The Silence of the Body

•

"The sun rose and the cry seized them," says the *Al Hijr* sura, because Sodom must be destroyed at dawn (sura of Hud 81, which derives from Genesis 19:23: "The sun was risen upon the earth"). *Saika*: cry (of the angel Gabriel) or rumbling. And the *ababil* birds shower the city with *siggil*, fire and brimstone. Medical historians (Sprengel, Hammer) demolish the myth, interpreting the fire and brimstone as smallpox. If Sodom was destroyed by smallpox, the vision of a city not only depopulated but burnt by a boil, stone by stone, would make a great Epic. Leopardi would have admired this visionary metamorphosis of an exploded pustule into fire and brimstone carried by "clouds of birds" ("Elephant"). In "The Smallpox Vaccine," Parini also sees it as "the furies of atrocious hail" and as "untamed, voracious fury" that "into the grave piles/endless generations of man." Yes, perhaps it was smallpox, seen as a sign of fire. Woe unto us, who, free from boils, are threatened from the sky by true tremendous fire.

•

According to John Keegan, the new explosive weapons have greatly increased potential suffering. Modern comfort must be paid for with war. We wish to avoid war at all costs, but at the same time we expand the peace apparatus enormously: Hubris. Production and Commerce in twin Belles Époques, diabolic facility of life, denial of death. To keep the balance, explosive weapons have to become ever more deadly: Nemesis demands this. Only a colossal famine would justify either a true disarmament or a decrease in the capacity of explosive weapons to balance Pleasure and Pain. The path we are following leads to tremendous wounds, to countless hospital wards reeling in pain.

•

A visitor to London in 1862, after seeing a Doss House for sailors, recalls a missionary's extraordinary description of another public dormitory, in Peking, called the House of Chicken Feathers. It was a huge dormitory, entirely covered with a thick layer of chicken feathers. The poor arrived by the thousands and made their nests in that ocean of feathers; at daybreak, they had to disappear, leaving a penny with the person in charge. (The price was the same for both children and adults.) In the early days, the owners used to distribute a blanket to each guest, but the blankets were almost never returned, so Chinese ingenuity found a way to reconcile philanthropy and sound management. A felt blanket the size of the whole dormitory was suspended from the ceiling by a system of cables. When the poor were tucked in to sleep, the pulleys lowered the blanket very slowly, like taps in the military, over the humanity submerged in the feathers. A number of holes allowed the guests to avoid suffocation by sticking their heads through; at the sound of the morning gong they had to be quickly withdrawn because the blanket was about to be pulled up. Beneath this fantastic canopy rising toward the ceiling, the raggedy multitude left the Chicken Feathers in an orderly fashion and went looking for some naked chickens.

•

"Life slips away from the brain and from the nerves . . . Modern nervousness is the cry of the organism fighting with the environment" (Rosolino Colella, *Nervosismo e civiltà*, 1905).

•

Onstage, while singing *Carmen*, on the night of June 2, 1875, the soprano Galli-Marié felt a sharp pain, as if a knife were stabbing her heart. She recovered and finished the act. She relates that in her dressing room, as she was racked with pain, she saw in a flash the pale face of Bizet. (Bizet died suddenly that night, in Bougival, a few hours after her vision.) The news of this premonition appeared in *L'Éclair* on September 24.

.

The state of Leonid Brezhnev's health. Western intelligence attributed various diseases to him: gout, leukemia, and emphysema. He wore a pacemaker. Yet he traveled, went to Germany for four days, made toasts, and delivered speeches against the neutron bomb, a weapon that disturbed him. An American newspaper said that he had a heavily drugged look about him, the effect of a steady stream of medication, and that he spoke with difficulty. He was escorted by a team of doctors: from Moscow he even brought his dentist and a cook, a specialist in his diet. In the building where he was staying, the German government had set up emergency services, with a sufficient dose of blood plasma and a pair of ambulances. There were enough German doctors at the disposal of the Russian leader to fill three Mercedes. Thus the last days of the master of the greatest totalitarian apparatus in history were prolonged by the relentless stranglehold of medical totalitarianism.

.

The misanthrope is, by necessity, the most strenuous denier of an anthropomorphic God.

.

According to a slightly confused Neo-Pythagorean theosophist, the Gorgons were the malarial fevers and Perseus the man who triumphed over them: the origins of the myth were Oscan, and in archaic Latin the Oscan people called the intermittent fevers *februe stakne* (from Stheno the Gorgon). I don't know, let me see . . . *febris* from *februare*, to purify, is possible, because a fever purges a man of an invading demon; deified, it becomes *Febris*, whose sanctuary today is a tiny glass rod containing mercury. The Gorgons lived on a rainy moor, amid gray statues of petrified men and beasts, many of whose faces, including our own, we would recognize if we were to pass through. More persuasive is the interpretation that makes the Stymphalian birds killed by Heracles—a multitude of bronze claws rising from the stagnant waters—symbols of malarial fevers (Robert Graves). There is a mythic affinity between the Stymphalian birds and the Koran's *ababil* birds, destroyers of Sodom: here fevers, there perhaps smallpox. (The idea of airborne diseases is rooted in the ancient soul.)

The mosquito is the only insect I persecute (though not with insecticides) to protect my sleep; but I let anopheline mosquitoes live, while I squash the *Culex*, which carries no plasmodia. I would let the poor creature suck my blood, but its whine makes me culicidal. Is it a crime to make such an ugly whine?

Herodotus says that Egypt was filled with nets: by day they caught fish; by night, stretched over beds, they warded off mosquitoes. In the weeks after the river overflowed its banks, there was a curfew in the Nile Valley. You couldn't leave home after twilight because the pools left by the flood drew endless legions of Stymphalian birds, whose parasites were ready to complete their cycle in human blood.

Malarial fever nails the invalid down: could the Gorgon's gaze have been malaria? Who can count the malarial zones in the world since ancient times? How many marshes and maremmas did Alcuin cross between Aachen and Rome before writing to Charlemagne: "My path is constantly assailed by an implacable brigand: Fever"? (There were no more temples to Febris: the Christians considered him a brigand.) Paludism

The Silence of the Body

sheds light on La Pia's memories: "Siena made and Maremma unmade me" (*Purgatory*, V, 134). La Pia was *unmade* by the implacable devastation of malaria; *made* (to live) by the pure, dry, clean air of Siena. Maremma is the infectious air, the corrupt climate, infested by the unmakers, Grassi's anopheline mosquitoes: *maculipennis, bifurcatus, claviger.* To truly understand Dante's line, imagine Siena, the way it still is today, and the bronze specters of the maremman Stymphalia of yesterday.

Puccinotti wondered whether it was dangerous to cross the Maremma by rail, but he found that the train's movement, smoke, etc., were excellent prophylactics for the traveler because they pierced the marsh's thick miasmatic veil. Before shooting the swamp birds with poisoned arrows, Heracles drove them away with a great clattering of bronze rattles (the most archaic antipyretic), like a clanging train in the plain between Livorno and Grosseto. Entire lifetimes were consecrated to mosquitoes by doctors hunting hematozoan in bodies as shadowy as gossamer nocturnal flowers. In the end the Englishman Ross and the Italian Grassi fell to insulting each other over who deserved the prize. (Grassi's *Note storiche sul modo di trasmissione della malaria*, reprinted in Pisa in 1967, is full of bitterness toward Ross.)

·

Qual è colui che sì presso ha 'l riprezzo
de la quartana, c'ha già l'unghie smorte,
*e triema tutto pur guardando 'l rezzo**
(*Inferno*, XVII, 85–87)

Burning with fever, Dante traveled the malarial roads from Venice to Ravenna. He died in mid-September, when the

---

* Like the man who feels the chill / of the quartan fever, his nails already pale, / the mere sight of a glade makes him tremble.

plasmodial parasite is at the peak of its development. (The malaria season begins in March and culminates in September and is marked in Greece by the propitiatory festivities in honor of Asklepios: Asklepiades, Epidauruses.) Perhaps when Dante wrote those verses he was already feeling the symptoms of the disease that would unmake him as they did La Pia. Deathly pale, anemic as a lamp without oil, his fingernails colorless, the feverish Dante polished the *Paradiso* in his last days, burning and shivering. Under heavy blankets, amid the constant chattering of his teeth, the final visions of the journey were born. Perhaps the fever, like an epileptic aura, helped him to see God.

In an article dated November 5, 1948, the Vatican newspaper proclaimed its jubilation over the new Heracles of the sixth labor: DDT, which had been in use for only a few years. (Before, they used to spray burning kerosene into swamps to get rid of anopheline mosquitoes: practices were already drastic.) Forty years ago, no one had even the faintest idea of DDT's consequences for the environment and for man (mankind is always blind when it undertakes something). The article only hints at the possibility that certain *Anopheles* (I was pleased to learn) resist DDT. In fact, when the most powerful anophelicides were tested, they failed to fulfill the utopia of total extinction but masterfully poisoned the malarial and the nonmalarial alike. Our chemical destroyers of parasites are neither rattles nor a hero's arrows: they are a chemical machine of planetary destruction. The anophelic doctrine is in harmony with myth and demonology: just pull a secret lever and these two distant cherubs appear at its sides. Such a beautiful, strange mosquito is almost supernatural . . .

There are too many petrified heads for the Gorgons' activities to have been limited to a single man confined to his bed by fever. Giovanni Verga is the magical recounter of the malarial epic: "Malaria seeps into your bones with the bread you eat, and if you open your mouth to speak while walking down the street suffocating in the dust and sunlight, you feel your knees give way, or you sink into the saddle of your mule ambling along with its head down." In "Malaria," a short story of infinite beauty, the true Gorgon appears: "It seizes the inhabitants from the empty streets and nails them to the thresholds of their homes, whose plaster is crumbling from the sun; they shiver with fever under their brown cloaks, with all the bedcovers around their shoulders." Verga was a malariologist without peer, and he did not care in the least that Laveran had already caught plasmodium by the tail a few years earlier; his style thrives on the inexplicable fatalities, which etiology knows only as the actions of obscure powers. Lake of Lentini, plain of Stymphalia . . . The Heracles of Verga's wretched sufferers is quinine sulphate and eucalyptus tea, and Sulphate-Eucalyptus battles the bronze-clawed birds in a sixth labor without end.

·

It is right to close the insane asylums. We have finally realized, but refuse to acknowledge, that everything human compressed inside the walls of the world is insane asylum: houses, cities, gardens, temples, fountains, cars, theaters, passions, laws, necropolises, diseases and health, parliaments and prisons, universities, brothels, and churches. Like all other insane asylums, this planetary asylum has its lights, its do-gooders, its kind deeds, its doctors, as well as its tormented souls and its incurable killers. There has never been a shortage of melancholiacs in power, of paranoiacs leading huge crowds. Unfortunately, this is an asylum we cannot close or even improve. The overcrowded cells should worry the director: anything could happen in them.

Since man is a cancer, his metastasis on other planets should no longer seem so improbable.

.

In the darkness you were searching for a hand: you found an ass; its big cow breath warms you; you find twenty other hands.

.

"I protect the cow, and the spider too." But what if they ask you about mosquitoes? about microbes you started exterminating before you were born?

.

The senatorial oligarchy was no good, but Catiline was worse. The *vir probus* could choose only the old order. With the senators he could negotiate; Catiline would have torn him to pieces.

.

In Sonnino, an almost vertical stone canal zigzagging between the houses (apparently no different from the others) is called the Alley of Pleasure.

.

Cunnilinctus. We haven't heard the final word on cunnilingus: it's time we did. Essentially, I will present cunnilingus as one of the philanthropic acts that provokes the least ingratitude. (*Fellatio* lives at the window across the way: whatever can be said about her holds true to a large extent, but not entirely, for him.) The entry in the *Dictionarium Eroticum* starts right out with some philological nonsense: *Foedistas* (foulness) . . .

The Silence of the Body

The Romans were great practitioners of cunnilingus. Poets and philosophers disapproved of it but did not abstain from practicing it. Their disapproval was meant to defend the virile toga, to defend the free man from a servile act, but it no longer concerns us, because we no longer wear togas (outfits brimming with connotations of disapproval and prohibition). Today the distinction between free and servile acts has been blurred, and a more complicated and paradoxical moral can choose servitude as freedom. (There is Christianity here too: a teacher, Jesus, *washes* the feet of his disciples, making an example of himself; a messiah dies on the cross, as a slave; therefore in the Christian ethic the free man can perform cunnilingus.)

But cunnilingus undoubtedly has a servile past; it was the sexual act of eunuchs and of seraglios, the desperate pleasure of imprisoned women. Today the harmony of conjugal relations rests, illicitly, more on cunnilingus than on any other act. " '*Señor*,' said a Spanish lady to a gallant, 'en el medio está la mejor estacion,' as if to tell him that he could kiss her middle as well as her feet and hands" (Brantôme, *Vies des dames galantes*). Women who refuse it show a kind of anti-Kama impiety, an irreligiousness in the erotic sphere. The main risk of cunnilingus is forgetting the person on whom it is performed, since the act immerses the devoted practitioner in pure *Shakti*, in the immortal sign of the Mother, in the infinite waters of Maya. Sunken in the symbol, swallowed by the waters, the lover loses sight of the woman's face and name. When she discovers this oblivion, this work of Cosmic Energy (in the middle of her Comb, every woman has an eye that sees all), her human ego is wounded. Prolonging the act increases the risk. Everyone has felt *elsewhere* during prolonged cunnilingus (like Narada, when she goes to fetch water for Vishnu), in an unknown landscape, wondering, "Where am I? Why am I here? How much time has gone by?" Face and name, place and time are lost.

With *fellatio*, this does not happen. The fellator does not travel in the indefinite and passive; she is tied to an active pole, and the act is confined to a very short period. The penis acts as a compass, the fixed North of the ego (a symbol, but also too much the individual wagon wheel to plunge into Maya). The face is nearer and hangs lovingly over the mouth that sucks.

Whoever practices cunnilingus must try never to lose contact with the human and the individual, because the divine overwhelms and obscures, however one encounters it. One must do everything possible, interrupting oneself every so often, to keep memory alive—with words, glances, and caresses—so as never to leave the small personal orbit. One must never isolate oneself! The masters say to let the woman receiving cunnilingus set the rhythm with her movements, assuming the best positions to draw the secret energy to herself. (The tongue, purveyor of the word, is infinitely more powerful and energizing than the penis.) A Sade would not understand. If lewd egotism, monstrous and unchecked, befouls the mystic immersion, strips of its philanthropy the arduous caress that excites rapture, cunnilingus becomes one of the many mirrors reflecting our filthy image.

A rigorous and esoteric transcendence would condemn cunnilingus as excessive enthrallment to creation, offensive to a transcendent, speaking God. Remember your Creator . . . Remember me and I will remember you . . . Difficult to remember, in those moments. (Jews and Muslims are restrained by the indirect image, Christians by the severe *gaze of the cross.*) To care for plague victims *in God's name*, until you yourself die from the plague, will not corrupt transcendence; but cunnilingus in God's name appears foreign and contrary to religious vocation.

What was the *sideratio*, the *sideris percussio*, the astral thunderbolt: punishment of the lickers regardless of their other merits? Martial wrote an outrageous epigram about Nanneius, *moechus ore*, lover with his mouth (XI, 61), that kills any desire for *lingere cunnum*:

> *nam dum tumenti mersus haeret in vulva*
> *et vagientes intus audit infantes*
> *partem gulosam solvit indecens morbus.* *

The hypothesis that the *indecens morbus*, "shameful disease," is a hardened chancre is disproved by the *dum*: Nanneius is struck at that very moment. But the tongue is weak; exertion and acidity can cause sudden allergic reactions (better known to the ancients than to us), including *sideratio*.

In ages when *Mal des Ardents* was widespread, oral intimacy often planted the distressing signs of *Treponema* inside our poor mouths. "The mucous membranes of the mouth and of the tongue, thin and well vascularized, lend themselves marvelously well to penetration by *Treponema*" (Jérémie Vilensky, *Chancre syphilitique de la langue*, 1930). Saliva is a swift messenger, and the sinister nummular seal especially favors the front third of the tongue: the upper part, the edges, and the tip. (Cunnilingus is only one of many means of contagion: in the nineteenth century glass workers frequently got ulcers in their mouths from using the same blowpipe.)

The sublime watercolor illustrations to the *Atlas der Syphilis und der venerischen Krankheiten* (1898), by the celebrated Viennese physician Franz Mracek, include a particularly horrendous *Sklerosis labii inferioris oris* (figure 8), which shows no *harter Schanker* on the tongue (I don't think I spotted one when I leafed through). But figures 3 and 4 of Vilensky's

---

* For, so long as, having plunged in, he remains stuck in the swollen vulva and hears the infants within squalling, a shameful disease paralyzes his gluttonous member.

work depict an ulcer in the middle of an outstretched tongue that resembles an extraordinary ocular globe with its pupil in the center, made even more strange and lewd by a mustache canopy hanging down on the sides. If this is what *indecens morbus* means, then the case of Nanneius could not have been better illustrated.

Sideratio could also be sudden paralysis as punishment for excesses (it was believed to afflict lovers intent on devouring each other's genitals). In the *Priapea* there is a *hapax legomenon*: the cunt is called *bait*, food and nourishment for the performer of *cunnilingus*; and so it is. Ode 78 alludes to a strange *sideratio*: a girl *fortis ante nec mendax*—strong before and not mendacious—is so badly afflicted in the *landica* (mysterious word for clitoris) that she can barely walk. A recent translator, Cesare Vivaldi, imagines that her *landica* is swollen, hard as a bicycle tire, but the text is not specific. There is no reason to imagine infection, because infection would not stop a woman from walking; maybe it was divine punishment.

Like all other acts, cunnilingus is white, black, black and white, neither white nor black; the prism varies from conjugal affection and erotic philanthropy to self-destructive lewdness. Cunnilingus on a streetwalker is already a death wish. Of all the acts in the lover's manual, cunnilingus is the most exhausting and melancholy, alleviated only by the joy imparted. At times, the lover turns melancholy before it's over; its incandescent fervor fades little by little in a cold dissipation of desire, and all that remains is a galley slave's arm tied to an oar and an oar mechanically stroking the impassive ocean. Cunnilingus fights bravely against Frigidity, which nevertheless increases and sadly envelops us. Thus you re-emerge from the crypts of an impersonal God without having been able to kindle a spark of joy in the mystery of a living soul.

The Silence of the Body

Laisse-moi, parmi l'herbe claire,
Boire les gouttes de rosée
Dont la fleur tendre est arrosée. *

Without drinking those "drops of dew" (better than the brutal bait of antiquity), you cannot attain a perfect knowledge of womanhood; any other knowledge is a colorless teaching, imparted in the damp shadows. You can know woman in the abstract, but to know an individual woman you must always grope in the dark, lick at her locked doors, and turn the keys that open a series of empty rooms. If you can guess anything it's a miracle. Do not deprive yourself of cunnilingus, lest you diminish what little light you have to lead you, fearless, into the human inferno. But remember your Creator in the days of your youth.

.

Leopardi's intellectual tragedy lies mainly in his horror of Enlightenment reason, which held and horrified him (he could see its future consequences), in his powerlessness to banish it (the darkness banished by that abhorred light floated in and around the Leopardi mansion). Giacomo suffered ferociously in this vise. He knew that "reason is the cause of barbarity" (only a mystic or an absolute reactionary could have dared to say this), and in his attraction to opposite sympathies, he felt *unfit* to do battle with reason. Landscape and the music of poetry as Leopardian flight from rationalist barbarity, from that tormented place. It rains, the birds sing. There is a truce, an escape.

.

* Let me, amid the shiny grass, / Drink the drops of dew / Sprinkled over the tender flower.

It was customary to remove the flesh from the bodies of knights who had died far from their homeland by boiling them in water and wine, or in water alone. The cooked, melted flesh was buried on the spot, and the bones were transported home. (This was done to Barbarossa, who died between Larande and Seleucia in 1190.) Bone of knight, your arms await you.

·

In England, Napoleon may have been portrayed the way medieval artists imagined the elephant. In a beautiful caricature by Rowlandson, "Napoleon and Death after the Allied Victory in 1814," Death is seated on a cannon, staring into the eyes of Napoleon, who stares back. Here Napoleon is thin, with a long head and a mustache. The magic of his abhorred name is enough to evoke him.

·

Hippocrates says that a disease in which sleep is painful is fatal, while one in which sleep provides relief is not. With laudanum, morphine, and barbiturates, we have lost sight of this distinction.

·

In the *Logia Agrapha*, Jesus says, "What white teeth!" about a horrible, putrefied dog. Four days after his death my father's face was already unrecognizable, but his hands were perfect and white, and passing through that underground crypt, Jesus would have said, "What beautiful hands!" This is salvation.

·

In Seveso. Everything seems normal, yet there is a plague. On July 10 the chemical boil explodes. The forbidden zone is poorly guarded, and anyone can pass through by avoiding the main roads. The children play and ride their bikes to the edges of the most contaminated spot. In the stores a sign guarantees that the produce comes from elsewhere. Rain has fallen on the first posters put out by the Health Commission, which said not to be alarmed. ICMESA is a huge iron tumor over Meda, which borders on Seveso, a silent dragon at the center of a meadow covered with its own slime. This is how, if our eyes were not sealed by a spell, we should see Industry, which everybody desperately, wretchedly adores. Industry is a mythological animal that deals out death, a Minotaur to which everything must be sacrificed. Tomatoes and lettuce ripen in the gardens, untouchable. The sky is heavy and filled with fumes. A region in the grip of industries, where disfigured lives persevere, in an almost unreal ugliness, chronically ill and bandaged. The power of Man: the toxic cloud killed the animals but (for the time being) only sprayed acne on the children of man (August 26, 1976).

.

Dr. Richard Blackmore asked Sydenham what authors he should read in order to become a good physician. Sydenham recommended Cervantes.

.

On a moving train I was running away from an evil, ambiguous man, maybe a vampire, and our suitcases were open, abandoned.

.

A struggle between two concepts. In 1917, the prevention of venereal disease among the troops was so important to the United States government and high command that they restricted individual freedom and interfered in the Allied countries. The British were more tolerant of *Treponema* and would not curtail the soldiers' freedom to get infected. The moralists in England did not want people to even talk about the fight against venereal disease: their enemy was vice. But not even the preachers demanded the suppression of brothels: the virtuous soldier was expected to spontaneously refrain.

.

If you have a bell near your bed and know that no one will come to your assistance, you are in the ideal condition to need God.

.

An enormous scorpion crawled through the house with the wagging motion of a female mammal feeling pleasure. I went to get a glass to trap it, and it disappeared. In its place there had sprouted a mushroom with eyes and a bird's beak, but alive only as a plant, and a beautiful insect, a kind of peacock-insect with long wings, was sucking on its head. I put the glass over this strange natural entity and sat there looking at it. Artemidorus says that dreaming of scorpions means an encounter with evil men.

.

For Stendhal stubbornness can be a sign of genius; for Montaigne it is the clearest sign of stupidity. But stubbornness, by itself, merely indicates the presence of energy in a neutral state. In addition to or in lieu of something else, it becomes a sign.

.

"God himself generates guilt in mankind when he wishes to completely destroy a family" (Aeschylus, *Niobe* fragment).

The Silence of the Body

What do we have to feel guilty over? Over being—all of us —viscera that can be penetrated by guilt, continuously impregnated with guilt by someone who wants to destroy us?

.

In the police handbook for the states of Parma and Piacenza, dated October 14, 1815, one article orders the police to keep an eye on, above all, "vagrant madmen and dangerous animals." The author of the regulations must have been thinking of Psalm 59.

.

Unexpected affinities: Ludovico Ariosto and Confucius. They are connected by a weak, mysterious thread: their common birth in Virgo. The *Orlando Furioso* can be seen as a perfectly performed traditional Ritual, an act of obedience and Confucian respect toward masters and fathers. One can also examine Ariosto's and Confucius's relationships with other men, full of ceremonious fear and tedious precautions. Confucius served as governor for Duke Ting and for the Duke of Lu; Ludovico served as governor of Garfagnana for the d'Este family. Confucius said, "If men endowed with goodness were to govern for one hundred years, they could eliminate infamy and abolish the death penalty." Ariosto wrote: "I naïvely confess that I am not a man to govern other men, because I have too much compassion, and I do not have the effrontery to refuse anything that is requested of me."

All Ludovico needed was "a little cowmeat and mutton," indifferently cooked. Confucius wanted well-cooked meat, finely chopped, but in small quantities, never more than the rice. He drank a lot of wine and spurred his intelligence by seasoning his food with ginger. Out-of-season fruit horrified him (as it does all Oriental diets). And he never spoke while eating or while lying in bed. Silence at the table is a supreme maxim. Collectors of Table Talk are analeptics of impurity. Compare Confucius's silence at the table with Luther's verbosity. Luther's constant chattering was extraordinary testimony, with powerful belches, but there is no true wisdom to be found there. It is more like grumbling by blind Nature, the mute foaming of an earthquake. Confucius's silence is much more magisterial. All the sinister coarseness and madness of great Christianity amid jets of saliva, jawboning of badly cooked cow, spiced pig, beer and St. Paul, grace and sausages: fascinating and grandiose, but keep away from the Maelström. A tiny piece of Confucius's ginger contains the peacefulness of a truly sapiential landscape.

When I am not forced to speak while I eat, I too am relaxed and happy. How can you put up with people who gather at mealtimes to cross spoons and idiocies and who, while eating, discuss, gesticulate, fight, talk about things that happened, make business decisions, critique books, and convict or acquit defendants? It is a torture to be avoided if you are not like them. I would agree to eat in company provided no one breathed and a beautiful calm voice read things that were easy to digest.

·

More afraid of female domination than of the Great Fire, the Puritans dreaded the eschatological coming of the Whore of the Apocalypse. But that strange Whore is both male and female, neither female nor male; it is a city, the City, power of iron and stone, handcuffs and mental flight: *your* City too, Puritans! In the depths of life, perhaps there has always been female domination: what happens on the surface is not very important. We see a petrified world: the contemporary world is a giant paralytic who does not invoke the thaumaturge because it fools itself into thinking that it is running toward the abyss, when instead it is being pushed, rolled, and kicked

The Silence of the Body

in that direction. Like machine-gun bullets, men, women, and everyone simply submit to the movement thrust on them. I had hoped for a revolution of Maenads, for a bacchante's riot against the iron city, but a few shouts in a public square is not even good theater. The prevailing authority among women will always belong to those who for the sole sake of giving birth let their ova be robbed or themselves be injected with the semen of dead husbands.

.

In his portrait of Machiavelli, Santi di Tito created something new in demonological painting. He worked not from the model but from a precise notion of Machiavellian fiendishness. As a picture of Intelligence whose Heart has been removed, his Machiavelli is a true demon of the future.

.

Evacuating you can think of life and death; eating you can think of everything; in orgasm you think only of nothingness. It is a mystical emptying, but for everyone.

.

"Thus when you present for our inspection a girl whose external genitals are hard, solid, shiny, and a rosy color, with nicely joined labia majora, tiny, covered labia minora, a short clitoris with its prepuce, vaginal folds that are prominent and contiguous to each other, deep mucous sinuses, a narrow vaginal opening and uterovaginal duct, and the hymen in its state of integrity, we will say quite readily that these are the signs of physical virginity" (from an elegant lesson in forensic medicine, Francesco Puccinotti's *Della verginità e dello stupro*).

.

It would seem that women take greater risks shoplifting in department stores and supermarkets during their menstrual period. This attenuates and may explain their stealing: they are evidently moved by a need for caresses.

.

A knowledge with no clear idea of Evil as universe and principle, a knowledge that pays no mind to the evil that man is and was and for which he is forced to atone, is a knowledge with a view to Evil, in favor of Evil, and probably suggested by Evil.

.

A good doctor must go beyond the notion of Good as Life and Health, and Evil as Death and Disease, because such an overly professional horizon will stifle his moral life. If his moral life is not sufficiently broad, he will be unable to truly understand life-health-death-disease and will never adequately comfort his patients. His actions must always stay inside that schema; but his thoughts should rupture and rearrange it, so that his actions are soft and light, not monotonous and servile.

.

El honguillo viene por sí mismo—The mushroom grows by itself—say the fungi-eating Indians, and the rose blooms without any reason, says Silesius. But what about man? A little Jonah, he carries the huge whale of Fate in his stomach across the mad sea of the world, where the mushroom and the rose grow without reason.

.

"What is this stuff?"
"The DNA of an Austrian corporal from the Great War,

son of Klara and Alois Hitler, named Adolf. It's the key to everything."

"The key to what? To decipher a genetic code, like any other biological information or human gesture, I need a word that pierces the darkness. Then I'll try to fumble around on my own."

"Choose: Fate, Zeus, Angra-Mainyu, God, Predestination, Karma, Anunnaki, Moira, Sin, Mystery, Evil . . ."

"Thank you. Each of these skeleton keys is good. Naturally they're not enough, but each instantly supersedes the previous one, which is left behind as if it had been struck by lightning. The reading of the ulterior darkness will be adapted to the eyes' ability."

·

The flying hornet and the crocodile's mouth are the emblem of Crime and of everything harmful (*Horapollon* II, 22). I walk around Rome, Milan, or Paris: I run into swarms of hornets, and everywhere crocodile mouths open wide.

·

Sexual love in degenerates and criminals is the flip side of anatomic and physiological knowledge: it is analytic, dismembering, and shattering. It gets you nowhere; essentially it is the wrong approach. Psychology, like Psyche, behaves just as criminally, with remarkable maniacal excesses, but the discovery of its victims, piled high inside books, does not lead to judicial inquiries. (Only a few great artists have managed to keep Psyche whole and alive when they *dissected* her; the scientific psychologist is completely incapable of such miracles.) But infinite love does not analyze; it cloaks beauty and pain, and all the misery of the flesh, in its mantle of compassion; with feeling it sketches on our clothes the faint outlines of the ever new drawing of absolute Unity, the

furthest point from the rational divisions that bring us closer
to murderous practices.

.

The Mantis is called *praying* because of the kneeling position
of its hind legs, which snatch and kill while praying. But
doesn't a praying man also behave like a mantis? With groping
arms he tries to catch and devour God. The attempt almost
always fails, but our instinct is theophagous.

.

Julien Benda wrote: "Phaedra feels not the slightest ten-
derness toward Hippolytus. If he were ill, she wouldn't make
him a cup of tea. Now that is a woman truly in love." No
Racinian lover would make a cup of tea for an ailing Hippolytus. Perhaps this is what fills the objects of their passions
with such panic. No man wishes to be the object of murderous
passions, not even a hero; the warrior wants his wounds to
be dressed. All of us look on our lover as a night nurse, a
hand to soothe our agony. Knowing that we are *mortal*, we
imagine, wishfully, that woman is not and yearn for the
bandages of her mysterious, nonmortal condition.

.

Catherine of Siena saw blood as a drug: "Therefore, it is quite
true that he is a physician, since he donated his blood as
medicine" ("A Prigioni il Giovedì Santo in Siena," *Episto-
lario*).

.

And she saw blood as even more than a drug. To Queen
Joanna the Mad she wrote: "But in no way can man's appetite
be sated or his thirst slaked save with blood." Who was Catherine of Siena in reality? What chthonic waters surfaced in

the mirror of Fontebranda? She would not have been so immensely intoxicated by the mystical blood of the Word had she not been just as intoxicated by the smell of human blood, the basis for the comparison.

.

Every day, behind fragile shelters all over the earth, part of humanity sheds blood from an obscure wound. The Moon is the killer.

.

In the *Coloquio de los perros* Cervantes absolves the witch of children's blood: "The unguent that we witches rub into ourselves is made from extremely cold herbal juice, and not, as common folk say, from the blood of babies whom we drown." Into the unguent went a pharmaceutical arsenal with a disinterested purpose: to procure an encounter with *the other God*, without her undergoing physical death and a judgment that would condemn her to an opposite good. Belladonna, black henbane, mandrake root, thorn apple, poppy, solanum nigrum, aconite, hellebore, and hemlock (honest excipients: lard, fat from a hanged man). Surrounded by black fumes, the witch oils the entire surface of her body, trying to make the magic unguent penetrate as deep within her rectum and vagina as possible. Did she realize that it was easier for a drug to be absorbed through the internal passages?

We do not know the witches' lore, only their desires. The alkaloids (atropine, scopolamine, morphine) in their unguents and the muscarine in their mushrooms had unknown properties. But their religious aim, their desire to see the horned God and to make him their own, helped their nerves absorb the hallucinogenic substances, and in that excited frenzy everything became possible. Their fingers rubbed layers of horrifying greasy paste into their greedy orifices.

Faster, faster, *emen-etan*, to the witch's sabbath, to the Great Appointment!

One explanation for *Membrum et semen diaboli frigida sicut glacies* (The devil's member and semen are as cold as ice): the unguent was made from *extremely cold* herbal juices, and when the witch lovingly pressed it inside, she already felt possessed by the God. Thus with self-induced suffering she discovered that member and spermatic fire were *sicut glacies*. Even the broomstick, the witch's flying rod, was rubbed with unguent, and its touch was equally cold. But all did not end in toxic delirium in a smoke-filled room: Margaret Murray describes actual witches' sabbaths in the forests, real ceremonies in honor of the A-Christian God, the deposed gods, a desperate liturgy of the defeated . . . Without ritual, they would remind us of the poor's drug parties: deprived, senseless, and lay, not heterotheistic. Only in the sad glimmer of a persecuted dream of the transcendent does the witch's sacrifice become meaningful and not just pitiful. Unfortunately, oiled inside and out with formidable alkaloids, they were easily forced to make horrendous confessions and brought upon themselves the punishment of their religious enemy, the crucified Protagonist who kept vigil over his cities and fortresses.

·

"Theories of vice contain something more thoughtful, profound, and true, something that does not appear in vulgar and often inexact expressions of responsible maxims: in this way perversion can easily appear to be a logical progression" (Manzoni, *Fermo e Lucia*). This is the purest, most apotropaic comment possible on Sade's black illuminism, as if Manzoni were issuing a meditated response from his Brusuglio home to the phantom of the Bastille and of Charenton, from his orderly rows of mulberry trees to the ardent chaos of prisons and asylums. A virtuous man might have included the perfect commentary in a handwritten epigraph to the letters of Aline and Valcour.

.

Duo sunt praecipui fontes e quibus manant omnes litteratorum calamitates, mentis assiduus labor, corporis continua requies; quantum etenim mente et cerebro negotiosi tantum corpore otiosi —There are two main sources from which all the troubles of men of letters spring—the mind's assiduous labor and the body's constant repose; in fact, their minds and brains are as busy as their bodies are idle (Tissot, *De Valetudine litteratorum*, 1766). In the past two centuries, almost everyone has been afflicted by the ailments of the literati: *Et alvinas foeces et urinam diutius comprimunt ne turbentur labores sui*—They retain their feces and urine too long, so as not to disturb their work. (Georges Valensin wrote: *Aujourd'hui l'urination est réglementée sauvagement chez les civilisés*—Today urination is savagely regulated among the civilized.) They suffer from bad digestion: *Qui enim cogitat intensius . . . cibos ingestos coquit difficilius tardiusque*—In effect, whoever reflects too intensely . . . digests food more slowly and with more difficulty (while imbeciles *multum quotidie comedere, perfecte tamen digerere*— eat a great deal every day yet have perfect digestion). The perpetual *fluidi nervei dissipatio*—dissipation of nervous fluids, causes infirmity and mental illness. Tissot describes the case of one young man *bonae spei, qui de quandrando circulo anxie nimis sollicitus, delirus in nosocomio parisiensi obiit*—of great hopes but who, too anxiously preoccupied by the squaring of a circle, died delirious in a Paris insane asylum.

All food that is *pinguia, viscida, flatibus turgida, natura aut arte durata*—fat, oily, flatulent, and hardened by nature or artifice—is bad for writers. No legumes, no fava beans . . . Onions, a flatulent food, would not be recommended, yet they are a symbol of the Sun, an Apollonian food . . . *Levis sint coenna*—Dinner should be light. Agreed. Tissot issues an astounding warning: *Pestiferus enim labor mox post pastum* —Working right after meals is destructive. Not only destructive but unproductive: *Dum tumet ventriculus mens languore afficitur suisque deficit muneribus*—When the stomach is full, the spirit is stricken with inertia and becomes deficient in its tasks. Naturally he recommends *accurata masticatio*, careful chewing. Raw eggs, well-baked bread, aromatic condiments: thyme, marjoram, salt, nutmeg, cinnamon. Drink a glass of cold water as soon as you rise. Take one hour of postprandial siesta. *Lenta est alimentum coctio in doctis ventribus*—Food is digested slowly in the learned man's stomach. A golden maxim: *Nihil est quod non possit accurata dietae institutio*—There is nothing that a carefully organized regimen cannot do.

Tissot praises the virtues of chocolate but violently attacks tea, and this pains me: *E potibus litteratis amatis detestanda est in primis infusio famosi illius folioli, thee dicunt, quod in perniciem nostram quotannis, retro iam duo saecula, ex Sina et Japonia advehitur*—Of the drinks loved by men of letters, the most despicable is the infusion of that infamous little leaf called tea, which to our detriment have been imported from China and Japan every year for more than two centuries now. It destroys the nerves—*Totius corporis robur subvertit* . . . He prefers coffee! (Provided it is taken, like wine, *pro rimedio non pro potu*—as medicine, not as a drink.) He describes the harmfulness of tobacco (*cephalagias, vertigines, anxietatem, lethargum, apoplexiam*) and mentions that Francis Bacon compared it to black henbane and opium because of its effects on the brain. To relax the stomach, he recommends massaging it with coarse wool in the morning before eating, while lying in bed with knees bent. Avoid bathing in hot water: *Prosunt frigidae lavationes*—Cold baths are good for you.

"It is true that if a man of letters, indefatigable in his

studies, adopts a balanced diet, innocent and frugal, he will find the discomforts of his profession more bearable" (Felici, *Dissertazioni*). Sitting is the great malady (*culpa sessionis*), but perhaps since I have been on my feet too much, I now suffer from bad circulation. At least two hours a day of *ambulatio*. Madame de Sévigné wrote: *Je suis persuadée que la plupart de nos maux viennent d'avoir le cul sur la selle*—I am convinced that most of our ills come from keeping our asses on chairs.

·

Morgagni writes that in the morning, if he obsessed over some abstruse subject before rising, his nose instantly began to bleed (*De Sedibus et causis morborum*).

·

Priapus essentially means father. Its Egyptian origin is noble: *Fre-Ab* (or *Ap*), Father God or Father Sun (Lanci, *Lettre sur les hiéroglyphes égyptiens*). In Hebrew (from which the Greek noun derives): *peri-av*, father of the fruit. But we cannot use *priapic* or *priapean* as synonyms for *paternal*; they are synonyms only in the silent depths of the word.

·

"How could man, in the perversion of his senses, dull his instincts to such an extent as to make them accept one of the most toxic products in the vegetable kingdom; and how could Nature fail to perform its task, how could it demean itself so much as to allow man to obtain pleasure from the smoke emitted by the combustion of this deadly plant, tobacco?" (Maurice Phusis, "La Chute de l'Humanité," *Biologiste*, 1920).

·

St. Augustine was fascinated by the spider capturing flies; Spinoza used to deliberately feed flies to the spider. In that

161

moment, where were the Philosopher-Saint and the Saint-Philosopher?

.

The death penalty could be replaced by public damnation, a compensatory ceremony that feigned bloodlessness. Performed well, with real fervor and a good crowd, it could effectively ward off both present and future crime. The same sentence could also be passed on unknown individuals, who thenceforth would never feel safe, anywhere, from its consequences. After a while, some victims of the curse would surely die. People would call their deaths a coincidence, of course, but a hardly negligible goal would still be achieved: the establishment of a magnificent terror. "May he be cursed by day, cursed by night . . . may he be cursed by the air, the day, the night, the beasts, and the children." The most dreaded disease would be summoned against him: a slow, painful death, God's law of retribution, the *lex talionis.*

Occult proscription is terrifying. Kill in effigy; the criminal will not laugh. If the effigy does him no harm, it will help him, forcing him to atone by killing himself or struggling to make amends at grave risk. (A challenge to rationalists: Since you consider malediction innocuous, why not allow it? It would be only a game. If you forbid it, you will have succumbed to the unknown.)

.

Julien Sorel is magnificent: "J'ai voulu tuer, je dois être tué—I wanted to kill, I must be killed." This is the noble murderer, the man who even in his guilt never ceases to be fair. If the author of even the most heinous crime speaks thus, he was only momentarily lost and has found himself again. But the adversity we must endure is another: the multiplication of criminals completely unwilling to give up their lives in atonement for the lives they took. Not one day in prison will they accept, and their friends are ready to kill other people to prevent the service of that minimum of justice still attached to their prison sentences. Julien's words are divine. There is something terribly disheartening about a contemptible felon refusing all punishment. What can be done for us, for those he has killed, and for him? We know he will end up winning, that his fear of atonement will restore his freedom and that in a certain sense he is already *free* when he refuses his sentence. By the same token the man who accepts his sentence, or wants a greater one, has in a certain sense already seen justice served.

.

In his *Plan de législation criminelle*, Marat vigorously opposed the death penalty. If such a bloodthirsty man favored abolishing capital punishment, then someone of opposite beliefs could legitimately spill blood in support of it.

.

Fortunately, the U.S.S.R. was a power without justice. Its perfect, radical absence of justice was a parasitic worm, the profound cause of the colossus's breakup.

.

The *shewa* is unpronounceable because it signifies "nothing"; it is the vowel of silence. But the mobile *shewa na* is pronounced by a special divine dispensation to voice that Nothingness.

.

Peace between two nations does not exclude a general war of mankind against all, a perfect cycle that naturally includes

163

mankind. Therefore, the peacetime we live in is an endless seething of wars that spare nothing, scorching and overpowering everyone.

．

In our sleep, we try to cry for help but cannot emit a sound: the dream can only vent our fear in a choked, interior hoarseness. Distressed over the consequences of the technological growth of nations, all we can squeeze out are faint sounds that none can hear. Even if many of us were to shout, all together, we would not produce a universal cry that could be heard by humankind as it sleepwalks toward the fire. We are crying out in our sleep.

．

"Nevermore shall I be a murderer," says Society, under the weight of her infamous old justice and the scourge of humanitarians. "Here is a sword," say Ate and Ananke. "Now you must die." But Society is also horrified by the suicide sword. "Either kill or kill yourself," reply Ate and Ananke, implacable. Society begins to run from room to room, and each room that witnesses her rejection of all decision fills with confusion and screaming, with senseless deaths, and with fish roasted on pikes by violent men, while carnivorous stars stick out their tongues from the windows, swelling with human poison to spew out in silence.

In the last room the shades of those who died without justice pounce on the frightened woman, shove her against the wall, and slit her throat. Society too becomes a grieving shade: "My God, if only I had dared! If I had only struck dead whoever it was that knifed me, spilling innocent blood! Why didn't I do it? Why *cecidere manus*, did my hands drop? This story's conclusion is not simply a moral, like "fight for life"; it is the immorality of Society's suicidal refusal to per-

The Silence of the Body

form legal executions. This secret flaw generates the visible disorder, the irresistible demand for bloody punishment that infects the tree from top to roots. If Punishment completely disappeared from the system, there would be no talk of slow death: Fall and Annihilation would be instantaneous.

.

Aportez moi un orinal/Et je verrai dedens le mal (Bring me a chamber pot/And in it I'll see what you've got, *Le Roman de Renart*). This is what the fabliau says to poke fun at doctors, but could they really see anything? It cannot be easy to derive an exact diagnosis from a chamber pot unless one has authentic powers of divination. Analysis with the naked eye requires a well-honed skill. To *look* at urine requires the same ability and power as to diagnose with the iris. Everyone knows that an ugly color is a bad sign, but only the Great Medicine Man can determine what disease it indicates. It is nice to imagine the pensive faces concentrating on the yellow liquid that symbolizes the Mystery of the Waters and that of Human Health, the finger that samples, the nose that sniffs, the moist lips that part to deliver the verdict.

.

If Money is a symbol of Excrement, greed is only a form of coprophagy. (The molten gold that the Parthians poured into the mouth of Crassus probably signified excrement, but only the red-hot symbol could act as his executioner.)

.

Altdorfer's *The Daughters of Lot* (Kunsthistorisches Museum, Vienna) shows a Lot who is anything but pious—indeed, he is extremely, gluttonously lecherous. Maybe *he* got his daughters drunk, because drunk (and old), he couldn't have done much. Here you can see the Bible's force, its willfulness.

165

When the Scriptures decide to save someone, they do so, constructing and guarding the person with a sword of pious, *zaddiq*, perfect fire; they proceed in this manner with many others. These specially protected figures, whom we would tend to see among the sinners—headed by Cain—bear the true mark of election.

.

Why do the evening papers scream so loud? Why do they exaggerate everything? Why do they love blood so much? Because they belong to the *evening*, and they rub the day's events into the diseased back of the Night. Some of the impending darkness enters the print shop and guides the hand that sets the headlines. After a quick perusal, the evening papers are thrown away with a certain revulsion.

.

Harriet Martineau said that in Baltimore the bodies of white men were never used for dissection (*Retrospect of Western Travel*, 1838). Black men did not like serving anatomy either, but as slaves they could not refuse their bodies to science.

.

Petronius's amazing maxim *Medicus enim nihil aliud est quam animi consolatio* (For a doctor is nothing more than consolation for the spirit) reduces medical practice to its essence— psychology—and equates medicine with landscape, poetry, perfumes, and love (Seleucus' speech, *Satyricon*, 42).

.

"Man is just a drop of sperm" Yes, but *Gutta cavat lapidem* —The drop hollows the stone.

.

The Silence of the Body

"Prayer is a healing," said Muhammed, according to al-Bukhari. What he said is profound: it is a healing, which is much more exact than *it heals*. Prayer cannot heal, but *it is a healing*; it does not give health, it *is* health. Immediately one senses the refreshing breath of greatness.

.

A Japanese proverb says that a man who likes carrots also likes women. This can be put to the test by suddenly setting a plate of carrots in front of a homosexual.

.

According to a macrobiotician, chewing fortifies the sexual organs because they are connected to the jaw muscles (an Oriental teaching). In voracious, hasty chewers, one can observe a degree of impotence. This connection is quite plausible, since we are dealing with a single hunger.

.

A society that treats murderers as if they were mentally ill or unhappy souls in need of treatment will only end up exasperating them. After providing the best proof of their destructive urges, they are denied their actual dangerousness, prevented from being somebody, and insulted by the offer to construct something! Those who dare to destroy yearn profoundly and especially for their own destruction. Reason mercilessly refuses their wish. Murderers step up their efforts, like drowning men asking for help or buried miners beating against solid rock. "Please, answer, give us death!" Opponents of capital punishment always give the same response: "Go ahead, drench the world with blood, you will still live."

.

Genesis says that man is but flesh alone, meaning that man is only weakness and suffering. But *flesh* also means cluster of cells, density of atoms, aggregate of chemicals. If man were flesh alone he would not even be weakness and suffering; he would be less than nothing. Without being explicit, the same book that teaches *he is but flesh alone* also taught—solely through the miracle of dogged reading accompanied by the thirst for transcendence—that our flesh is the involucrum of an imprisoned spirit, sentenced to prison but not to death.

.

In Naumburg Rudolf Steiner saw Nietzsche, who by that time was raving mad. His spirit-soul entity, Steiner said, was all but gone, held to his body only as if by a thick rope. It was as though the real Nietzsche were hovering over his own head. Steiner saw Nietzsche as the reincarnation of a Franciscan friar who had practiced intense self-mortification. In Nietzsche's earthly life, that mortified soul was reluctant to be immersed in the corporeal and material. Zarathustra as the fruit of a deadly struggle between Minorite ascetic and Naumburg philologist. (Steiner appears in Kafka's *Diaries*: the clairvoyant theosophist as seen by the Prague scrutinizer of souls.)

.

Hitler was also a Malthusian, but the remedy he proposed was not philanthropic. Instead of birth control, rapacious war and extermination of other populations.

.

In his *Treatise on Acute Diseases*, Hippocrates says: "Being born and dying are the same thing; mixing and separating are the same thing; birth and mixing are the same thing; perishing, decreasing, and separating are the same thing."

In reality man is made for more and cannot bear the marriage bond for long without becoming despondent. Too much mixing with woman is harmful. Love with excessive mixing—its greatest degree of perfection—is noxious. We were made for the plow, the hunt, war, poetry, music, God. Filled with rooms, landings, photographs, elevators, conflicts, worries over responsibilities, we are exhausted into imbecility. We do a little erudite research as if we were embarking on a voyage to the Trojan wars, to Lepanto, or to conquer Peru.

·

We are creatures of glaring frailty and puniness, lost in a discomforting galaxy, at whom the gods threw an anatomic knife, along with harps and grains of wheat, so as to see inside the sacks forsaken by their breath before consigning us to earth or to fire. What did I do? I caught my fingers in the harp; from the grains and knife I received perfume and nostalgia. But well-sharpened and squeezed, the harp becomes a knife and also a healing juice. I cannot call myself either doctor or usurper.

·

If the cadaver were not sacred, it would not contaminate your hands. Its impurity was prescribed as a sign.

·

Decision comes at night, a fragment by Philo suggests. So Night is the one who decides. Behold the darkness at the helm of history.

·

When the fatal illness appears I hope to be conscious and helped to see it clearly; the problem will be how to resist, how to avoid treatment without too much natural suffering. Disease is less frightening if one reflects on it. The endless exams, therapies, and the whole medical apparatus do not reassure me; they distress me. I will fight for power rather than calmly offer my flank to an ointment. The most urgent problem will be finding a doctor, not a cure.

.

Paul Valéry's response to the final disease—"Je suis foutu et je m'en fous—I'm damned and I don't give a damn"—remains the best possible (even a religious spirit can find it exemplary). To be perfectly wise without ceasing to be human, pronounce the first part firmly (realization of the ineluctable fact: "Je suis foutu!" Good! You're right!) and the second part with secret reluctance, a slight hesitation, to spare one's human reality from trembling at the prospect of a loss one fears complete—that of everything the unsaved person believes him or herself to be. On close reflection, Valéry's response also suits nations, empires, religions, civilizations, and the whole of humankind—every apparition of matter.

.

The tigress suddenly appeared in the bedroom, where we were sitting at the table eating. She was very calm, but her presence banished all tranquillity. Though respectful of books and other things, she brushed against a row of bottles and glass jars in the hall, then smashed them with a few swipes of her paw, without hurting herself in the least. From that moment on we grew truly terrified, as if the broken glass represented our wounded flesh.

.

The Silence of the Body

Weimann-Prokop's *Atlas médico-légal* observes that fly larvae can completely destroy a cadaver in a few days. They paint it when they destroy it, making it assume the strange appearance of a figure from a very non-academic portrait. In layman's words, a hideous sight. Is this decomposition a demon's outrage at a house that a pure heart has abandoned or a kind of postmortem pillory, the true, hidden features of the deceased soul finally emerging in the light of day? One day we shall all decompose—a thought we do wrong to stave off—but not everyone decomposes publicly, with the participation of mice, ants, and flies. Public decomposition could become an exemplary display, a sign of punishment. Those who decompose openly, however, are almost always the unfortunate, the lonely, suicides whom no one cuts down from the rafters, old people who had already purged their sins through too long a life. Every death carries the sign of fate's absurd futility.

.

For the second time in a few months, my right knee came out of its socket and left me disjointed and in pain, anxiously awaiting its return. Perhaps it is a werewolf, off to howl in some countryside, devouring sheep or children. Afterward, behind a bush, it gets dressed as a right knee again and comes home hanging its head. But like a mother I wait up apprehensively each time. What if it never returns? Right now, in bed, my knee far away, my leg in a vise, I fear it will never return.

.

A pain in my leg, my brain races and thinks: Leg leg leg. It becomes all leg. Ditto if the stomach, abdomen, or bladder aches. The brain is a supremely mimetic organ. It imitates so well you could mistake it for the intestines, for the bladder

. . . but when the brain gets sick, it does not think *brain*; it is ashamed to show itself as it is, an offstage actor, an ordinary man leaving by the stage door.

.

Female frigidity is a *memento mori*. Man wanders through a sepulchral darkness, stumbles into a pile of bones, and gets a whiff of inscribed marble. Kohelet must have known the beds of many frigid women to dictate, in the furor of profound experience, *Mar mimavet haishah* (More bitter than death the woman). Frigidity and *frigor mortis* are related. This general maxim could be derived from the huge numbers of frigid women throughout time. Woman is not death because of sin; she is death because of her glacial absence in the beds of love. Rare furies and beautiful angels frolic through this desert of salt and ice: they are the true female Erotic Temperaments, animators of life, of romance, and of poetry. Yet female erotic ardor and passionate rapture are deceiving: they give man the illusion of immortality and transport him, stupefied, to otherworldly places. Female intelligence has created the proper means of transport, the *ne quid nimis*: erotic pretending, the art of making man believe that the ice is boiling. Hence the geisha practices the supreme female art, the foundation for an authentic female education. Frigidity and ardor are distracting. Something is missing from both: in the psychological sense, something too depressing or exhilarating; in the Gnostic sense, something whose voyage of initiation does not terminate in the light (the frigid woman abandons you in the darkness) or begins badly, casting you headlong into bedazzlements that confound the ways of knowledge.

.

Carnal people desire a God whom they can touch, at least with their reason. They get what they deserve; God remains intangible. He is the *mistater, al-batin, absconditus* God, the God who makes spiritual people vibrate like lutes unforsaken by sound. *Adoro te devote latens deitas*—I adore you devoutly, O hidden Divinity . . .

.

I wondered whether the so-called Black Holes at the heart of the galaxies—the closest one, thirty thousand light-years away, with a diameter of many millions of kilometers, has been spotted in the constellation of the Swan—might be an astrophysical version of the Gnostic vision of the Realm of Darkness. It is not a question of comparing texts; they are two separate languages, two unrelated speculations. All stars could turn into Black Holes when they die, expanding the Realm of Darkness. It would not be compact but made up of enormous, immobile, scattered banks. Thus the destiny of Light would be ultimately to reenter darkness. Behold the macro- and the microcosms. As the star becomes a Black Hole, so does man return to dust and shadow. A Black Hole is heralded by the storms of gravitational waves and X-ray emissions that indicate swallowed matter (it feeds on stars), but it does not emit its own signals. It is a silent black *object*, a dead mass that has increase, not life.

Giordano Bruno saw all celestial bodies as large animals that hurl their excrement into infinite space. He would consider the Black Hole a big carnivore absurdly deprived of an excretory canal. The vampire sucks blood but does not excrete. Has anyone ever seen vampire urine? The Black Hole swallows matter without returning it; it does not metabolize; it is a stellar vampire.

The Manichean *Epistula Fundamenti* describes an Earth of Darkness that exists alongside the Earth of Light: *Erat tenebrarum terra profunda et immensa magnitudine, in qua habitabant ignea corpora, genera scilicet pestifera. Hic infinitae tenebrae ex eadem manantes natura inaestimabiles cum propriis fetibus; ultra quas erant aquae caenosae ac turbidae cum suis inhabitatoribus; quarum interius venti horribiles ac vehementes cum suo principe et genitoribus."*

Like the Realm of Darkness, the Black Hole is photophagous. Like a spider sitting behind a luminous body, it draws the body toward it when the moment arrives and the light dies. But the Manichean Earth of Darkness is a Black Hole where much life is concentrated, life of horrible substance and color, yet still legitimate life. The astrophysicists' Black Hole suggests more the idea (a strangely *luminous* idea) of non-being, or rather of no-longer-being. Their Black Hole could be the antimythic Realm of Darkness, the true Land of the Dead:

> *Le sépulchre solide où gît tout ce qui nuit*
> *Et l'avare silence et la massive nuit.*

> *The solid sepulcher wherein all harm dwells*
> *With miserly silence and the massive night.*

We are approaching certain visions of an a-Satanic hell that is neither cold nor hot, that is harder, more stifling, and certainly more realistic. But the Pseudo-Dionysius the Areopagite rejoices: the Black Hole seems deliberately crafted to provide him with an objective image of God's Nothingness, of the Nothing-God preferred by his negative theology. The Black Hole would be his symbol and not the Ark, because the divine Nothing is also here, amid our cerebral labyrinths

* "It was a deep, immense Earth of Darkness, inhabited by a destructive breed of fiery bodies. In this place was infinite darkness, emanating from Nature itself, inestimable with its own progeny; there were also muddy, turbid waters with their own inhabitants; and in the midst of them, horrible and violent winds, with their leader and progenitors."

of streets keyed to the perpetual rumbling of sewers, here in our bodies that emanate light and spew urine and feces. The difference is that our symbolic Nothing returns the probes sent into its finitude.

·

War heals the wounds of peace by making its patients die en masse.

·

Where there is no atonement for crime, the tragic becomes a fermented poultice, a suffocating cloud. Zola takes the place of Sophocles. The tragic can regain oxygen and light only by fully accepting moral responsibility again.

·

While reading Speer's diaries, I thought about how the two most demonic personalities of the century, Lenin and Hitler, evaporated into nothing, even if one became a pharaoh in a mausoleum and the other disappeared in a gas explosion. I find the third demon, Stalin, inferior to the first two in the chthonic hierarchy, despite his enormous ferocity. He resembled too many other sadists in history. He did not create a new darkness . . .

Lenin and Hitler actually seem to have performed their task thoroughly. All that remains, all recollections of them, are fictions and disguises, antiques, reflections, leftovers. No one would dare call himself a *Hitlerite* today; the death of the man canceled out the demon. Lenin, by contrast, did not die on January 21, 1924. His life as a perverse shade has been exhausted only toward the end of this century. Although in twenty or thirty years there may still be little groups of henchmen familiar with his name, adopting it in self-justification, the period of his occult action has ended. The Russian empire regenerated by Lenin could survive or fall without *Leninism*'s having any significance to the ruling Beast-Party. When the Spanish Communist Party emerged from underground, it sought to be *normal*, eliminating the demon's head. Erich Fromm analyzes Hitler as an example of necrophilia with a long, fiery tail. Lenin needed a Dostoevsky. To prevent him from ever returning, imagine him as a Russian Jacobin. There are no more Jacobins.

·

My veins bother me, especially at twilight. I will digress on veins. The *libido coeundi* is born from the veins, according to the Chinese translation of a Manichean treatise quoted by Puech. In the City of Veins, the demon of lust imprisons the light force and plants the tree of death, of Dark Reflection. From Dark Reflection is born the libido, and from the libido the hapless Human Generations. In Latin, the veins are the seat of the life force, or the life force itself: *Deficient inopem venae te*—You are helpless and your veins fail you (you have no energy, you are exhausted; this is a Horatian physician speaking, *Satires* II, 3, 153). The wicked swelling of the veins revealed the Vein of Veins in the rising Penis, and satiric, priapic language uses *vena* as a synonym for *mentula* (prick). (Corominas refers to the meaning of "vein" in Castillian argot as nerve, tendon, muscle.)

   The Hebrew word *orqim* does not distinguish between sinew, arteries, and veins. In Job 30:17, *orqim* are rodents, because sinew, arteries, and veins *do not sleep* while they gnaw at the sick. (The Septuagint translates *orqim* as *neura*.) The Manichean treatise uses "veins" to refer to blood, in accordance with the classic biblical identification of blood with the life-breath (Deuteronomy 12:23: *dam* is *nefesh*). Meister Eckhart interprets a passage in John to say that blood signifies everything in man that is not subject to his will. So for Eckhart blood could refer to blind natural will, the libido unhindered by being and procreating.

Fabre d'Olivet interprets *dam* as everything that assimilates and becomes homogeneous, everything that is confused with something else, the idea of that which ceases to be different, which identifies with everything, which placates itself and sleeps (*La Langue hébraïque restituée*). Fabre understands *nefesh* in a spiritual sense: if blood is *nefesh*, it is both material and spiritual, blood and soul, vehicle and bond. (He does not see the tree of death.)

.

A heraldic angel appears and proclaims: "The threat of nuclear destruction and overpopulation (which are closely connected) will be lifted from the human race, provided that everyone gives up aspirin and dental anesthesia. Remember: this is a very modest price to pay for banishing from your midst the specters of Fire and Hunger, from which you will otherwise find no escape!" The governments are perplexed, so they declare a public referendum. I already know the result.

.

Meister Eckhart gives three reasons why a sick man refuses to pray to God to heal him (and implicitly deny the religion of the Psalms). A God full of love could not tolerate his illness unless He had good reasons for wanting him ill. If God wishes the man to be ill, the man must not wish to be healthy. Finally, it is not right to pray to such a great and powerful God over such a small matter: it would be like traveling a great distance to see the Pope and, once granted an audience, asking him for a fava bean. If everyone were so ashamed of asking heaven for fava beans, prayer would completely disappear from the world. Much has already disappeared, because today people are asking for all kinds of cures and salvation from the world, not from heaven.

.

It is right to feel jealousy and nostalgia in the face of the great spiritual despotism that makes people say, Hey, you, don't waste time burying your father, follow me. You should feel the same way about the charismatic leader's absolute power over life and death, though you must suppress any precautions and reservations that might seem to diminish it. That power made General Pancho Villa kill the wife and daughter of Tiburcio Maya point-blank, because Maya had said, I can't come, I have to think of them. (The evangelical commandment *Let the dead bury the dead* and this bloody episode from the Mexican revolution share a similar ruthlessness.)

We feel this way about birds' wings, predators' flight, and any sublime power hidden in human beings. But from those whom we love and protect we obtain even the smallest favors only with a lavish expenditure of *please*s, *if you don't mind*s, *can I ask you for a favor*s, *thank you*s, and *sorry*s, all uttered in the subtlest tones. We hear our children rebut us with "I haven't got time." (And not because they have to bury us— or, perhaps, because they do!) We are humiliated by our failure to wrest from them, out of love for us or at least out of a practiced feeling of devotion, that sputum of time we would be denied even if we assumed a more commanding tone. All because we are lacking the inner cudgel. Sometimes we have merit, the basis for authority, but merit is useless if we have no inner cudgel.

.

Too many bundles of nerves touching each other, too many threads knotted in a living tangle in the human labyrinth;

The Silence of the Body

you can hear the planetary dementia grow like the sound of the ocean. The earth has become a species of mononation, whose delirium, gestures, passions, and nightmares can be heard, seen, and foreseen everywhere. It is disheartening to think of this big, insane creature, from whom it is impossible to live apart; it occupies and usurps everything, sitting on all the chairs, grinding its jaws before every plate, its pockets filled with knives and an insatiable homicidal mania. Who can cure or stop it? What can a thinking person do? Avoid his fellow man? Found a colossal psychiatric empire? Many historical diseases have recently taken their leave of our suffering. But if life stays, suffering cannot go: it is a bald head changing wigs, and Death is ever present, the wagon, the scythe, the Landsknecht's bony hand caressing the Matron's fat pubis, Brueghel's *Triumph*.

The greatest merit of medicine's progress may lie not so much in its having tamed pandemics as in its having reduced male urological torment. Our overly long urethra, our alchemical bladder. The urological drama is still going strong, but it has shifted from Senecan-Elizabethan horror to more measured tones. (But sensitivity to pain has increased enormously, and this compensates for the decrease in suffering.) Kidneys-urethra-bladder: man carries his toolbox full of instruments of torture through the Fundamental regions. Lucky the man who urinates well until death. It is consoling to know that today no man has to die with the pains of Epicurus.

Meanwhile, a monstrous mushroom has sprouted in the areas of the planet where the most industry has gathered and the most life has concentrated. Environmental cancer is upon us and *in eo vivimus, movemur et sumus* (in him we live, are moved, and have our being). The chemical fires and the nuclear reaction produced in these areas, guarded by a madman, shedding their melancholy light on the universe—

for the future of medicine, these must give us pause. We will have to pour vocations and philanthropies into the perforated vessel of burns, radiation, and internal and external ulcers caused by technologies already out of our control at their birth. We will have enough congenital deformities caused by the ruined environment and wounded genes to fill thousands of sideshows. There will be little we can do against this scourge; the only prophylaxis is sterilization and abortion. We should teach future doctors about this and tell them, "You will have to face mysterious plagues and obscure pandemics caused not by fleas nourished on mice but by incandescent shards of human intelligence. The plagues of 529, 1348, and 1665 and the cholera of 1830 are memories, but you will witness more dramatic events, you will experience harsher, more painful hours."

In 1913 physicians and surgeons had no idea of the work awaiting them on future battlefields and in undernourished cities of women and children. One year later phosgene was used for the first time in Ypres. The rapid gangrenes gave the amputators no respite. In 1918 the Spanish influenza was the new cholera. After 1935, the novelty continued with fire, the drowning of cities in fire. Medicine had learned to save the wounded in the field, making amputations rare, but had Asclepius stared at the sky over a Japanese city on August 5, 1945, he would not have seen or imagined anything. And today we float on a sea of fire, waiting, on a single sea of silent fire . . .

We must apply refreshing bread to burns and multiply inventions to fight the hydra-headed aggression of fire. The fireman in every doctor must be awakened and kept at the ready. Not even one centimeter of burnt skin should be left without a coat of salve. I am obsessed by this thought, because after so many horrors, the great, incurable human madman continues to ignore the frailty of the flesh.

The Silence of the Body

·

The European escape from the world to other parts of the world: Samoa, Tahiti, Texas, and Ethiopia, by Meneliks, Tyroleans, Provençals, Andalusians, and Magna Graecians. All this is closed to us today. The cloud travels; everywhere the water is the same, the food is poisoned, ugliness and the need for money never cease to gnaw at you. Emigration is useless, except after an undesired political change or from an evil Russia. Two possible escapes remain: voluntary death or *spiritual* life. Never were so many doors closed in the visible. We can detect a sign: either the spiritual or death. Violently or gently, one can still escape *from* the world.

·

No matter how much justice there is in a city, the mere presence of slaughterhouses places a curse on it. However noble a medical research project may be, its experiments with live subjects will always place a curse on it.

·

Confucius says that in China the sale of fruit picked out of season was prohibited. (If the prohibition no longer stands today, then there truly was a revolution.) The profound good of such a decree completely escapes our societies, which have no spring or fall.

·

Calvin and the kidney stone. Tortured by colic and finally unable to bear the pain of retention any longer, Calvin, an old man (in 1563 he was fifty-four, which used to be old age), mounted a horse on his doctor's advice and rode, suffering horribly, until the shaking made the stone drop. On his return home, he pissed murky blood. But the next day the stone passed from his bladder to his urethra and with some hot compresses was finally expelled: it was as big as a hazelnut. A stream of blood followed. Thus God freed Calvin from the stone and gave it to the Genevans instead.

.

A gynecologist, Odette Poulain, expertly assessed the state of gynecology in 1967. A list of female torments before the antibiotic revolution: metritis, cervicitis, vulvovaginitis, salpingitis, salpingo-oophoritis, perimetriumitis and peritonitis with their complications, rectocolitis, urethritis, pyelonephritis, and phlebitis. For lack of rapid and suitable treatment, gynecological diseases were interminable, with long sojourns in bed and repeated surgery. Later, venereal diseases and puerperal infections. All, or almost all, the serious illnesses have disappeared, except cancer of the uterus, which oncologists consider one of cancer's finest specimens. After 1945, instead, the triumphal march of leukorrhea (white discharge), caused by *Trichomonas* and *Candida albicans*, a parasite and a fungus: troublesome and migratory, especially *Trichomonas*, but not serious.

Aristotle's "sick man" has become a healthy woman. Physical repugnance for gynecological diseases clearly underlies the moral invectives of misogynists: "I won't even mention certain disturbances peculiar to women, and their recurrence. Nothing is more disgusting to see or to smell . . . At the age when man is at the peak of his prowess, woman is already undone. Their soft, delicate, weak bodies, subject to serious disturbances and crushed by labor pains, quickly show the signs of aging" (Giovanni della Casa, *An uxor sit ducenda*).

With women restored to purity and health, the misogynist has no more fodder. Swift's Strephon can no longer find the chest of excrements and the explosion of vile things in Celia's dressing room; the shadow of foul mystery conceals the first bidet, deep as a grave. Balzac's aphorism "The husband who enters his wife's bathroom is either an imbecile or a philosopher" loses its meaning. An imbecile is an imbecile, even if he stays outside the door, and one hardly requires the *consolations* of philosophy to withstand the sight—hardly terrifying —of a woman urinating. (Whoever fears maleficent influences will, however, avoid crossing the bisected line formed by her open legs.)

Today menopause begins after fifty, but from the beginning the cycle is more unsettled. Cramps, amenorrhea . . . The fashion is to blame everything on folliculitis, while the ovarian sanctuary is assailed again and again by the bedlam outside, by the excessive trials the nerves must undergo to create and sustain contemporary existence and female freedom. But perhaps regularity never was a characteristic of these famous lunar periods. They are a strand of light that appears and disappears, a strange mirror that sometimes tells the truth, and sometimes lies and deceives. The ancient wound, the distant gnawing of fabled animals, was massively persecuted by hygiene and cosmetics to compensate for the curses and interdicts, almost a new face of man's terrors. Hence today the menstrual flow, provided it maintains a polite scarcity, is allowed to resist the specter of menopause much longer.

In Brantôme's day, menstruations must have been torrential: this intrepid soul compared them to a ram whose throat had just been cut. Today menstruation is a rivulet that dies instantly in a moor of asepsis. And the morbid men of Mea Shearim, in Jerusalem, are still afraid of an *impurity* reduced to a whisper, to an Aleph . . . They don't realize that skipped months are becoming more and more frequent! That gynecologists are unperturbed by amenorrhea! Moses could embrace any woman in all tranquillity, without first having checked her out . . .

Prehistory was completely amenorrheic. The woman of the future, the modern woman in whose eyes we will be ancient, may become amenorrheic, relieved of the heavy handiwork of parturition. These are signs beyond what we call history, but not messianic ones. True human history is inscribed in the era of this scarlet trickle, whose First Day's secret we will never know, since goodness and innocence are recognized only on the eve of their disappearance, after foul vituperations.

Today menstruation is praised, but the techniques for reducing and disguising it cast suspicion on this praise: we also praise the usefulness of the animal family at the same time as we destroy it. Menstruation bears the mark of the demiurge: it regulates female chaos and imprisons Tiamat in a twenty-eight-day cage. This may be why the Maenads' revolt employs the technology offered by the industrial demon to suppress menstruation and to liberate itself from *slavery* through inhibitors that suspend the cycle at will.

The image of the nonmenstruating woman is chaotic and could be as unrecognizable as the premenstrual woman of ten thousand years ago, who had enormous buttocks, with two pectoral breasts, two axillary breasts, and two inguinal breasts, or with a double row of four, as carnivorous animals have, and a milk capacity as durable as an oak tree. Perhaps in memory of so many breasts and so much milk, the matriarchy, in a correctly bimammary age, imposed itself on man, the eternal sucker. But with breasts reduced to almost nothing and babies nourished on powdered milk, a restoration of the matriarchy is impossible. The breasts would have to be increased to at least four through careful grafts.

Let us bless our good fortune: to live with women who still have breasts, who still nurse sometimes, and who still have living, though irregular, menstruations. The female mystery, however, has shifted from the shadowy regions that guarded it to the chasm of a disclosure at whose bottom the mystery will shatter. We were not supposed to know everything; not everybody deserves to know. The bottom of the chasm is inhabited mainly by the indifference that has crept into love and fear, and by a cautious dialogue that has replaced the almost absolute abandon with which Ibn Arabi said: After possessing a woman you must wash yourself, because you have been immersed in God.

.

Kafka wrote to Ottla from the Matliary sanatorium that he was sad "as a hyena" because he had given in to the temptation to eat sardines with potatoes and mayonnaise: he had once seen a hyena find a can of sardines, claw it open, and devour the cadavers. Only a true vegetarian could see sardines as cadavers and their can as a "tin coffin." A meat eater (I don't wish to write "carnivore," because man is not a carnivore) would not imagine he was cohabitating with chopped cadavers even if he was locked in the refrigerator of a butcher shop.

Non-vegetarians have a veil over their retina, almost a materialization of the veil over their soul, that prevents them from seeing the cadaver, the chunk of cooked cadaver, in a dish of meat or fish. In the West, almost everyone's eyes and hearts are blindfolded, but strangely, seeing cadavers is not the privilege of superior beings. Leonardo da Vinci, Tolstoy, Wagner, and Kafka were indeed such beings, but vegetarians do not generally boast superior eyesight. The case of Hitler deserves attention. Perhaps he became a vegetarian to imitate Wagner. More likely, he had a necrophilic visionary's *amor mortis intellectualis* (intellectual love of death) and was repelled by his mouth's material proximity to the necrophagic bait. Moreover, a demonic creature's eyesight cannot be inferior, in certain respects, to an angelic creature's. I am particularly soothed by the knowledge that Leonardo and Kafka were vegetarians. Uncontaminated, they traveled through a contaminated world carrying a light untainted by the grieving candles or dismal lamps of the slaughterhouse and the sacrificial stable.

In another letter to Ottla, Kafka mentions a bar of soap in his room whose scent everyone praises: "In my vanity I would have liked to explain the fact by my refusal to eat meat." Not eating meat definitely improves a person's smell, at least in life, and because of this and his great purity of heart Kafka must have been *myroblytês* (teeming with fragrance).

The desiccated body of St. Catherine, stripped of flesh inside and out, scattered fragrant sparks that smelled of lily, rose, and violet. But being vegetarian does not suffice: butter and cheese are bloodless meat, and eggs contain much meat, just as Caesar contains many Mariuses, and blood with excess salt and sugar gives off gloomy vapors. Bread is the child of yeast: it produces a bad smell. But nature is always ambiguous: garlic and the flatulent onion—great, necessary solar purifiers—generate heavy auras and gas; they contain sulphur (which is sacrificed to the gods) and an obscure drug that stirs the shadows of dreams. Olive oil, honey, rice, and tea are children of heaven. Bad odors couldn't possibly be born from such luminous foods.

The mushroom is a mystery: a mixture of light and matter. The individual's metabolism captures one or the other, depending on his or her prevailing inclination. (Vulgar people eat roast meat with mushrooms, thereby destroying the luminous molecules.) In a certain sense, eating mushrooms is cannibalistic, because the mushroom is somehow analogous to the human microcosm. Symbolic cannibalism can be good or bad, which is why so many precautions are required beyond the vulgar distinction between edible and poisonous. (Mycology, the study of mushrooms, is a sacred science.) The truffle is flesh of the earth, mummified cadaver, vegetable excrement, and stench factory.

.

St. Catherine does not consider any of the external and violent causes for the loss of one's eyes—a sign of times in which it was easy to be blinded by iron or fire.

.

In Turin, on via San Pietro in Vincoli, a quiet street that ends in a cemetery no longer open for burials. At twilight the sound of spoons and tin pans and the smell of hot food arose from the basement of one of the long buildings of the Cottolengo, making you almost wish you were confined there, the better to savor those sensations (pleasing only because you perceived them from outside). The noises were mixed with a kind of plaintive chorus, signals stemming from arrested brains set into motion by hunger, and with voices that gently issued orders and had a reassuring effect on those brains and on mine.

When not the fruit of inhuman architecture, and when limited in their dimensions, hospitals can impart the rare delights of warmth and human fragrance to patients and visitors. The great Theresian hospital of Vienna, Semmelweis's Golgotha, was gentle beneath the snow flecked with crows; perhaps another kind of gentleness was hidden behind its windows. The corridor and room of a maternity clinic on the third floor of an ordinary house where many years ago I visited a childhood friend who had just given birth seemed like bowls of angelic broth; I can still smell them. The smell of boiled potatoes, which at home is so vague, so indifferent, is comforting in a sick ward. And what a masterpiece of grace and human perfection was the gesture of the night nurse when she lifted the sheet to scrutinize affectionately a sad black trickle from the bladder of an old man whose tigerish prostate had been removed. There, amid an apparatus of tubes and glass where a carefully placed light slid steadily like a fake moon, she repeated her gesture at regular intervals, always with the same wisdom, without awakening the pain.

How many millennia, I thought, did it take for the female gesture to acquire such wonderful delicacy in lifting the sheet that covers a brutal wound! This gesture did not originate in the human female: it was created by time, which slowly transformed the gesture into woman: today you will lose three or four hairs and your nails will begin to reflect the almond and the fan, tomorrow your feeling for ornament will be born. A gesture that produced almost physical elation—like the caress of a trained Oriental courtesan who digs into your inertia to remind you of pleasure's duties.

Now, whatever happens, however ferocious the human world may be, a female hand whose slender veins hold all the *vis medendi* of the healing divinities, an eyebrow tenderly arched over the bloodiest wounds (how nice to fall asleep with this consoling thought) will always appear wherever there are beds, sheets, hemorrhages, and moaning.

.

Teach your sons and daughters the art of massage. It will be much more precious to them than your arrogant university learning. They were born into a time that has extreme and continuous need of it.

.

The index finger is related to the chest and the liver; the middle finger to the digestive system (especially the intestine), the spleen, the pancreas, the bones, and the ear. The ring finger is related to arterial circulation, the heart, the kidneys, and the eyes. The little finger is related to the bile duct, the nervous system, and the genital organs. The thumb is related to everything. A man who loses his index finger will have a smaller liver, and if the middle finger is lost, his virility will be lessened; the loss of the thumb weakens the will. All the internal organs will feel it if the whole hand is amputated.

The Silence of the Body

An alteration in the oxygen supply produces anomalies in the cells, making them anarchic and immediate targets for cancer. An analogy has been observed between the degeneration of these cells and the metamorphosis of cells taken from cadavers whose respiratory functions have ceased. Cancer, whose egg (hypothetically) is oxygen's altered metabolism, works to further lower cellular oxygenation, until the death of the patient, who already looks like a cadaver because he or she has been invaded by altered vampire cells (that make healthy cells similar to themselves by biting them).

The medullary relationship between cancer and industry may lie in the way factories steadily rob oxygen from everyone who works in them or lives nearby, and in the unstoppable and infinitely malignant proliferation of industry in the world. The oxygen exchange has become more exhausting for every aggregate of living matter (from coral to a brain cell, from a molecule of water to a gene). Industry closes the windows of life, one by one, and in exchange supplies rivers and oceans of anomalous money as monstrous as degenerate cells, absurd money that everyone grabs with enough rustle of paper to cover the sharp bang of windows closing. Our sticky-fingered efforts can never reopen them.

Monetary inflation is cancer, a cell without oxygen. Governments consent to the reduction of oxygen and the invasion of cancer by encouraging monetary circulation and industrial growth over the simple right to live and breathe. We are inside the mysterious, impregnable radius of a giant Cancer within which we frantically attempt to study and arrest particular types at the expense of an infinity of other living creatures. We can gather shocking proof of its oxygenophagia, but we have to pretend that it does not exist.

Money, the cancer maker and cancer victim, is spent *to*

stop cancer, a disease that is now tacitly recognized as epidemic. But isn't any contribution to cancer research by mortally wounded money ultimately favorable to the disease? This money is swallowed by the cancer-ridden pharmaceutical industry, a branch of the automobile industry, a twig of the steel industry, dependent on the uranium industry, mirror of the oil industry . . .

Revenues are used primarily for the maintenance, establishment, and expansion of industry, so every taxpayer adopts a fiscal alibi to help lengthen the Crab's claws. With the exception of outlaws or the poor (who pay no taxes), and of some surviving tribes (who ignore the glue-and-preservative industry), none of us can wash our hands of cancer cells. In this sense there is a collective responsibility for cancer's progress, and individual responsibility (the excuse that taxes are forced and involuntary does not wash) for manufacturing the cancer that afflicts our loved ones and neighbors. In the next room we can see the vampire stuck to their necks. They are powerless to push it away.

.

In an article in the *Journal de Paris* on April 27, 1792, André Chénier alluded to Robespierre as "a speaker noted for his savage dementia." A few words engrave an accurate portrait of him (this *is* Robespierre: lawyer, revolutionary, utopian), and the sign of the dark Beast who is coming, the Beast who will be a Demented, Savage Speaker in Robespierre's absence.

Behold Lenin, from the London congress to Smolny to the Comintern, leaden *parleur*, incarnation of the Russian furies and of Russian vengeance, monomaniacal prince of the most powerful materialistic Order in the world. Behold his loudspeaker, Trotsky, mouth always open, infectious and futile polemicist of an impossible eternal Bolshevism, the boot of new armies that will chop down all the birch trees in a liberated Russia and crush the red butterflies of Kronstadt. Behold Hitler, violent ectoplasm of the Brewery, Pythia of the beer cellars, millions of Robespierres in one frenetic throat. All exemplars of cosmic madness. (Stalin had the madness and the savagery but *he did not speak*: he was a silent monster, a true stone idol to blind, terrorized tribes.)

There are several minor monsters: D'Annunzio, Mussolini, Perón, Castro, Nasser, all the *parleurs* of the Spanish Civil War ("Amid rivers of blood, we are building a new Spain . . ."), but their oratory was greatly inferior to that of Robespierre, who had the advantage of a glacial mind uncorrupted by the phantoms of romanticism. The verbosity of contemporary popes is remarkable. They are good *parleurs*, whose *goodness* is infinitely suspect, because in the absolute absence of thought, pontifical goodness is an empty vessel, clean and neutral, in which one freely pours the foul sewage of ideas that guarantee the continuity of the satanic, of mediocre, banal opinions in which savage dementia ferments. Something connects the shade of that decapitated Jacobin to the Roman Catholic monarch, who massages the world using manuals of the most intolerable goodness. A dark film blurs their features behind appearances that make the comparison unthinkable.

•

Today medical school is attended by mobs, not students; a mob receives its degree, a Doctor-Mob practices the medical profession. We learn to distrust it immediately: this mob may even be armed, may even be equipped with powerful weapons. Whoever wishes to become a doctor should reflect before entering the profession; enter only if you are determined to be different and to adopt different principles and teachings. Otherwise do not enter. On the margins of omnipotent medicine, free spaces exist for Paracelsians and Neo-Mesmerics and for doctors armed only with Laennec's stethoscope or a few Chinese needles.

.

Delve a little deeper into a comparison of Pius XII and Hitler and you might make some interesting discoveries. Their relationship has a kind of symmetry and complementarity. The Pope's generic appeal to good and to peace was emptiness on display, and this void was exactly what the Hitlerosatan needed to spread unimpeded the dominion of his flags and work to the Catholic nations. Without nuptial pomp, in clandestine haste, the Pastor Angelicus welcomed the inferior word to his bosom, while forever simulating the insemination of the Word from above. He offered this Word the invaluable service of his silence. His mouth denounced evil as if it were *sine nomine* and did not bear those same sinister insignia.

At this point a formidable drama was grafted on that complicates everything but is good for historical chiaroscuro: the Pope gave the name of evil to the materialistic dialectic, without understanding (or wishing to understand) the Hitlerite anti-religion and its blood-dripping vessel of Providence dripping blood. Instead, he saw Hitlerism as the historical antithesis of the Soviet revolution and of the advent of Communism. The Pope immediately tended to favor Hitler as a good watchdog with a strong jaw, blessed, perhaps, with a pair of cherubic wings: he had neither the ability to see the presence of evil in both of the monstrosities he was summoned to judge nor the strength to use his two long hands to point simultaneously to both and say, "Gentlemen, behold Evil."

His obtuseness deserves to be called impiety. In such instances, a mediocre man situated in a high position is a sign that God wishes to destroy us. But in all fairness, Pius's reputation has been eaten away by censure. In his heart, the Pope made a sad, horrible *choice*. Suddenly, despite flutters of hesitation and superfluous verbal caution, all his prestige

The Silence of the Body

as a great religious leader plunged down the funnel of death planted in Hitler's barrel. Weren't his eyes opened by Bernanos, by Weil? No, the blind man would not allow a seeing person to be his guide. Thus he flung his anathema (which is essentially modest, like everything papal) at only one of the two monstrous faces, the one where it fell most ineffectively. The other face rejoiced, drunk on massacres, like Giles de Rais at Machecoul, and, with mouth ungagged, sprayed its infernal drooling over everything.

.

After eight hundred years, the sick have disappeared from the Pellegrinaio of Santa Maria della Scala, the Siena Hospital. What a sad impression one has now; with the sick there was life. I had been there a few years earlier at noon. The Pellegrinaio was swarming with cheerful old women popping out of the sheets to bring full spoons to their mouth and talk and shout about their fractured femurs. The fifteenth-century frescoes stretched their arms out over the white foaming of the beds, pulling them upward, into the painterly epic of time. Today the aseptic Pellegrinaio, after much traffic of caravans laden with infection, is a whitewashed sepulcher. For whom does the light from the enormous windows enter?

This is where the little nun from Fontebranda spent her evenings and nights. In my sleep I follow her memory from the dumbstruck room to the stone shard where she ended her brief night in the hard hands of God so as not to walk alone down via del Tiratoio—a street too dark and gloomy. Directly below the hospital vaults, off the beaten trail of the Catherinian itinerary, is the Chapel of St. Catherine of the Night. It is run by an order of Capucin monks, who offer prayers and services for the dead. The rooms are always closed, with a nice smell of catafalque, black cloth, and tattered paintings.

How did sweet Catherine care for the sick? In the Pellegrinaio of that time, nursing was everything. Catherine washed, applied balsam, bandaged, fed, purged, emptied chamber pots, and massaged. At times she might have ground medicines in the pharmacy. When her fingers squeezed a hand, her fluid spread through a body deformed by disease and reached the secret points of life that scientific medicine can touch only accidentally, and without much delicacy.

Compassionate and practical, she suppressed her transcendent impulses in the face of such misery. When someone spat up or lost blood or seethed in a coma, she resisted imparting the mystical commandments found in her letters: "And bathe yourselves in blood . . . and drown in blood . . . and sate yourselves with blood." These commandments were not for everyone, and to everything there is a season. But when she felt a patient was more *hers*, a nonrefractory, immediately catherinizable soul like Niccolò Tuldo or Neroccio Pagliaresi, then she brought out the cure of the infinite, the impossible medicine administered by angelic persuasion: rather than apply compresses and balsams, imitate the bloody rite of the cross amid the rags and pallets drenched with piss. She set her gaze on the temporal world and on a spiritual health most unhealthy for the body. She lived the harrowing Christian paradox: the best cure for the body is mercy; *spes unica*, the only hope, is the cross and death.

In the Christian world, every hospital was born as a projection of the cross, a vestibule of death. The French Revolution was the solar surgeon that placed hospitals in the service of life. (Now they hang in the void. They need death, they are refrigerators without death, dying without death.) Walking dreamlike amid the swearers and sighers, many of them feigning (Sienese *pícaros*), Catherine followed the insatiable Way of the Cross with an inimitable lightness in her step, moist with heavenly grace like a freshly sprouted mushroom. Familiar *mamma* of all that human wreckage, and infinitely *more*, living nipple given and multiplied, constellation without earthly measure. From her surroundings she absorbed the sperm of infectious diseases and pain, impregnating herself with it internally, externally, like a magic scapegoat. Then she withdrew into the tiny cell of the night chapel to sleep it off, flagellating her shredded temporal garment, drenching her habit and skin with streams of messianic blood that dried and comforted her.

But during the same epoch, a Chinese physician was certainly much better able to treat the sick than were the thin, sublime hands of Catherine, and with no less spirituality or wisdom. A patient at the Pellegrinaio was on the edge of madness, chance, and Christian insufficiency, before a landscape that was a joy to eyes that could see. Therapy must have been an unknown character.

The electrifying worshipper cast her material and spiritual comfort not at patients who might recover but at the agitated dust of bucket-kickers, condemned from the moment of their hospitalization to lose something, an arm or a life. The hopeless aroused her own powers of hope, which exhorted a perpetual healing in death. She lowered herself to change rotting bandages, in the invincible Christian conviction that it is better to have sores than to have none or be healed of them. In a certain sense, sickness was a beneficent interruption of sin and of blasphemy. (Difficult to understand such distant things; here I have set out mere conjectures and dreams.)

.

What if we had to choose to be in either of two places. The first is the Siena Pellegrinaio, with fourteenth-century illnesses and treatments (as well as its physical resistance to such cures), where we would be attended to every evening by St. Catherine, a unique creature and lofty spiritual magnet. The second is a modern, air-conditioned clinic, with late twentieth-century diseases and chemical and mechanical treatments, where we would be antiseptically assisted by two or three nurses paid well enough not to be saints and lacking both fluid and prayer. Who would choose Catherine? Not even the Pope would prefer the Pellegrinaio to his well-equipped Vatican clinic. There is nothing enticing about greatness, about a lone ray of greatness in the night, amid great misery and cold. An instant of communion with the transcendent, when one is surrounded by bedbugs and pus, can be enjoyed only under duress. But to Catherine's patients, her calm, the infinite calm emanating from her restless being, was her sublime gift.

.

Léon Daudet's literary memoirs (*Souvenirs littéraires*) contain excellent portraits of Charcot and his assistants at Salpetrière. I once leafed through his students' notes on his Tuesday public lectures: the most striking thing in his diagnoses of nervous illness was the absence of *sex* as a cause. (Freud would fill that void.) An interesting thought: "Medical, political, and literary materialism at the end of the nineteenth century in France was so perfectly foul that it convinced me, by contrast, of the excellence of those whom it had persecuted and of the loftiness of their ideals. The enemies of God led me back to God." (Led back, strangely, to a violently anti-Semitic God, who had Drumont for his Aaron.)

In my introduction to the Italian edition of Céline's *Semmelweis*, I did not include Daudet's extraordinary description of Péan, the surgeon in the Gervex painting that was reproduced in a famous Luna Park pavilion dedicated to the gynecological mysteries. This is how Péan operated: "After two hours of this activity, he was drenched in blood and sweat, with his hands—or rather, his clubs—as red as a murderer's, his feet dyed crimson, and he was always very cheerful . . .

This scientific massacre was at once butchershop, scaffold, and bullfight . . . Never had I seen such a mincemeat of human flesh, such a mountain of torsos, trunks, and stumps . . . His function in this world was to cut, open, resect, debone, and disembowel."

The master surgeon's temptation to put on a show has the same roots as a criminal's vanity; both men are pleased by their familiarity with blood and by their ability to taunt sacred retaliation. While the surgeon is encouraged by applause to multiply his challenges, the criminal inhales the incense he needs from newspaper stories about him. Daudet concludes aptly: "Nothing is more coarse and brusque than surgery when it is separated from medicine, when the person holding the knife does not realize that the knife is an extreme expedient, a defeat of therapeutic ingenuity."

.

From an alchemical text: "Open your mother's breast with a steel blade and penetrate down to the matrix." Jack the Ripper did this to the letter, taking five (or seven?) poor, hungry, sickly women as his mothers. He was driven by a shamefully alchemical need to grope through the *prime matter* and through universal chaos. He was not an adept; a purely symbolic descent into the heart of matter would not have attracted him. The parallelism is still striking: what the spiritual do figuratively, bloodlessly, experiencing and absorbing death in their being without giving it, was horribly, materially enacted by the mysterious murderer of 1888 on visible streets. Overcome by *nigredo* he ultimately sought peace in the black waters of a river, his final descent into chaos.

Poe's "Black Cat" also suggests images for metaphysical Ripperology. Jack opens the bodies to wall up inside them the Black Cat that obsesses him. The cat is still meowing on the streets of London, in the silence of the bodies.

Leibniz referred to Spinoza as a *physician* because in those days whoever excelled in philosophy was considered a physician or honored by the title. (Thus I will never be a physician.) Without attending the Anatomical Theaters and peering inside cadavers, a person was not really a philosopher. Rightfully so, because one must be a vulture before being an eagle, ready at every moment to turn into a worm, into an almost true demon, and turn back into an angel when the cock crows.

.

The Amsterdam ghetto swarmed with doctors. During Spinoza's youth, medicine was practiced by Joseph and Efraim Bueno, Abraham Farrar, Dionysius Benyamin Musafia, Isaac Vicente de Rocamora, Jacob Barrassa, Diego de Barros, Rafael Levi, Abraham Jessurun de Mercado, and Jacob Hebraeus Rosales, all of whom were Sephardim. The celebrated rabbis of Spinoza's yeshiva, Manasseh Ben Israel and Saul Levi Morteira, were nonpracticing doctors. At thirty, Spinoza had completed his studies of medicine and could teach it to Simone de Vries. Franciscus Van Den Enden, his Latin teacher, practiced medicine in Amsterdam and also taught it to Spinoza and to his other pupil, Kerckring, *vir anatomia pariter et chemia clarus*—a man equally famed in anatomy and chemistry (Van Haller). Frederick Ruysch lived in Voorburg from 1664 to 1666, a period when Spinoza was also there.

The most influential doctor in Spinoza's life may have been Nicholaas Peterszoon Tulp, the anatomist in the first of Rembrandt's two *Anatomy Lessons*; his works are in the Spinoza library at The Hague. In the village of Uwerkerk, near Amsterdam, the elderly Tulp was acquainted with the young Spinoza, who had just left the ghetto, and they spoke together about medicine, pharmacopeia, and philosophy. The mystery of Greatness touched Tulp twice, in his contacts with Rembrandt and with Spinoza. Both men witnessed his anatomical feats and were led to meditate on light and discover it in an obscure cadaver illuminated by Tulp's words. The contents and intentions of Spinoza's *Ethics* might, perhaps, be better described under the title *Medicine*.

·

When there is a *tremendum*, do not place too much trust in the faces and words of terror. Cancerophobia is required, but the most evolved humanity can be seen, spellbound, searching for cancer, a teaser being teased. And so it must be, because there is human adventure only so long as there is a craving for the abyss. What a pity that the vulgar miasmas of technical Hubris have replaced the epic and the tragic.

·

In a distressing dream, a woman with a retroflexed uterus sees a staircase whose top she cannot reach. The key symbolizes successful childbirth: it was customary to give keys to pregnant women. With the increase in cesareans, it no longer means anything.

·

In Brazil in 1930, some doctors maintained that cancer began to spread everywhere with the use of arsenobenzoyls.

·

Men harbored the suspicion, and the hope, that women were immortal. By a heroic effort, they were able to make sure childbirth stopped killing them. This made women *sicut Deae*, like goddesses, and drying out the old swamp of gynecological ills is an even bigger step toward female immortality. In the future, women will live two or three thousand years while men will go back to living thirty or forty years. Only baby girls will have some probability of seeing their mothers die.

.

In women, Giacomo Vercelloni of Asti explains, syphilitic ulcers in the throat indicate a *sympathy* between the throat and the vagina (*Traité des maladies qui arrivent aux parties génitales des deux sexes*, 1730). A Chinese gong sounds in the midst of the Asti countryside.

.

Bedsheets in the nations summoned to war in 1914 were drenched with semen, a great abundance of spermatic effusions. The young Hitler flooded his room with it in Munich, and in Zurich, Lenin's wife, Krupskaya, whispered to him, "Volodya, what's gotten into you?" War as a necessary detumescence. Sperm first, then blood, its son and father. Bedsheets, trenches, bedsheets. The armistice announced that the sperm was tired, the veins were empty.

.

Nemesis, disguised as crime, will strike painful blows against industry and industrialists. But why doesn't Nemesis use thunder or earthquakes? So that the punishment of the ignoble is ignoble, and performed by ignoble executioners.

.

I weep over all the destroyed breasts, all the excised uteruses, and wonder: Wasn't it possible to do something else, to forgo so much extermination, to avoid such infinite despair?

.

Elizabeth Wittelsbach, Empress of Austria, suffered from a *phobia of being looked at*. (She always hid from stares behind fans, parasols, and flight.) Her assassin stuck an ice pick in her heart without looking at her. Had she died amid lace and under canopies, the doctors would have made her suffer much more by looking into her face.

.

Somewhere among the classical and sacred texts I have amassed in my life must surely be hidden the secret of a special ecstasy, an authentic consolation capable of transforming the final struggle of the life forces, the hour of death, the final illness, the murmurs of a fatal wound into a moment of pure knowledge and of awaiting God. These books cannot simply be fortuitous choices opened every now and then and dusted off, inert spectators of agony intended merely to help promote *education*. They are actions, remedies, reparations, drugs, and active substances. They have their alkaloids to unleash and their healing elements to spring from behind bars. But who will guide my hand infallibly at the crucial moment? There will not be much time for browsing.

.

The crucifix in hospitals is not apotropaic; it is a symbol of the best Christian paradox. Through the obsessive presence of the crucifix, the Christians who invented the hospital attempted to radically deny its function as a place to restore patients to health and to normal life. The crucifix rejects medical therapy and surgery (although it shares a sympathy for the blood they spill), because surgery seeks to extirpate suffering and not to burn away, or even gnaw at, earthly pain. (Freed from a kidney stone or a fistula, a patient will seethe with even more sin than before.) Hence the sorrow, the profound misery of the hospital under that symbol for as long as hospitals were Christian.

The total secularization of life has made the hospital emerge as a place that can be calm and decent despite the negative presence of the crucified Christ, memento of the agony, the *Eli, Eli*, the *consummatum*, the ever-flowing hemorrhage. Now the symbol has almost completely disappeared except in hospitals run by religious orders, and its grand disappearance has left a void: the sense of death followed it into the bonfire, where it was *weakened* but not burned. A hospital filled with triumphant life and anti-Thanatos *pruderie* is no less gloomy (though much warmer and more pleasant) than a hospital dominated by chants of "dust into dust" and a bleeding rib cage. No hospital will ever be good.

.

"For without are dogs" says the last chapter of the Revelations of St. John the Divine with acrid Semitism, excluding from salvation all *molles, pédale, maricas del mundo*, faggots, perverts, endocrine chimeras, and gays, along with poisoners, the bloodthirsty, the foul, the sorcerers, idolaters, hardened liars, and impostors. *Without are dogs* is hard and brutal, snarling and fanatical; chains and burning stakes will follow close behind. Was Proust a dog? Was Cavafy a dog? Was Eisenstein? García Lorca? Lautréamont? Was Ser Brunetto a dog? (He wasn't for Dante.) Was Socrates a dog? Was Parmenides, Pindar, or Anacreon? Was Virgil a dog? What can save a salvation that condemns Virgil, since he too was a *dog*? Adopted as a prophet by the Christians, Virgil would be a dog according to Johannine rigor. The generic, anonymous category is always horrible. If you consider the verse's last word, loving and telling lies could lead to the exclusion of a sinner *contra naturam*, because he distorts the natural appearance established by law, but that is hardly sufficient cause to call someone a man-of-lies. He would have to have a completely inverted sense of the true and the just—which is the case with some people—but independently of any sexual fixation or activity. Sexual anomaly is only a somewhat negligible reflection of such an inversion.

The Silence of the Body

I do not like *without are dogs*. Discrimination becomes oner-
ous when one begins to talk about specific human realities,
situations, and persons.

·

Kafka's *Diaries* include a very simple phrase, almost a pun
on death that could indicate the extreme limit of the profundity man has reached in defining death: "an apparent end
that produces real suffering."

·

"Dreams can be defined as a brief madness, and madness as
a long dream" (Schopenhauer, *Essay on Spirit Seeing*).

·

Civilized people almost always repress their choler; failing to
expel it, they are poisoned by it (saliva also contains choler,
according to Bichat). We are all closed shops of repressed
choler (*repressed*, not actually controlled—swallowed with
great waste of precious nervous energy in order to stifle it);
what a sad sight.

·

"And thus the time that should be spent in reflection is
consumed in reading books with weariness of soul and body,
such that reading resembles the labors of a porter rather than
those of an educated man" (Guicciardini, *Ricordi*).

·

Self-control in the presence of living beings is among the
ceremonies said to be good and useful in the ninth edict on
the rock of Asoka. But our cities full of huge crowds and our
homes disfigured by human density rarely, and perhaps never,
know this good, useful ceremony. Cities are the place of
Repressed Choler, a kind of psychic waste that is not evac-

uated; many people cannot, ever, evacuate it. They push, turn red, strain, and groan: the choler hardens and does not come out. Other living creatures no longer have the pleasure of seeing a truly relaxed man.

.

When Disraeli was dying, the Queen's doctors refused him a consultation, since he had been under the care of a homeopathic doctor; their professional association rejected any contact with homeopathics. (On the Queen's insistence, they visited him.) The separation between the two medicines is still rigid. Today many patients have their illnesses diagnosed by ordinary doctors and then resort to homeopathic cures, an ark against the flood of poisonous therapies. This behavior reveals a twin distrust of both schools of medicine.

.

Tea and Garlic are equally divine, but Tea comes from God's *Sefirah Binah* (Understanding), Garlic from his *Din-Gevurah* (Justice-Power). Tea should be the drink of the good, the calm, the clairvoyant; but the wicked, the irascible, and the demented also drink it. One point in favor of God's moral neutrality. Garlic is a universal doctor, but many abhor his treatments; they refuse to be saved. Tea does not discriminate; Garlic does. Tea is delicious after one has eaten foods containing garlic, but it would be a fatal error to drink wine. The bad company of wine turns garlic into a killer, into barroom smoke. Anyone who mixes garlic and wine must be avoided, because he brings disorder and corruption.

.

Have only superficial relations with people who reject garlic and onions, because they have a weak character, incapable of profundity.

The Silence of the Body

•

Behold the twin conjugal cadaver slumbering on the white catafalque that saw how anxiously the cadaver attempted to separate from the Two and attain the inexpressible Oneness. But now each of the two sleeps, dreaming of waking as a divided fragment, as intoxicated with the illusion of division as it used to be—under the sign of love—with the illusion of undividedness. Husband and Wife are born from the decomposition of one flesh that used to be two different beings known only to gods or that acquire meaning only in the illusion that the world is real. Now they are rather ugly to see, sleeping in rooms preferably free of mirrors. In the dead of night you can hear the vibration of a mastication *mortuorum in tumulo* (in the crowd of the dead). One of the two, deceived by residues of shattered unity, caresses him or herself in solitude. This small separate ecstasy will not fulminate the individual; it will not make him or her die as biblical honey will. The individual will have to live in order to be transformed again, in order to completely savor the arcane decomposition from which he or she emerged with one free hand.

•

A surgeon boasts that he knows how to reduce the intestine by up to 90 percent. Bravo! Why not take away the remaining 10 percent: the Hunger monster would be gone forever.

•

No one contemplating suicide today would still choose sublimate—which made the gastroenteric tube scream in pain from fire in the pharynx and profuse diarrhea—and die after a few days of nephritis. Nor would anyone take a lethal dose of strychnine (five centigrams) and die in the throes of hallucinatory convulsions and tetanic contractions. Barbiturates offer an easy death, a sleep perhaps unburdened by nightmares. Another victory for the ordinary, for the escape from pain. This way one can leave by the golden gate, but where will one fall? A serious suicide chooses the Via Dolorosa, which allows the person to immediately atone for much of a deed that could be displeasing to God.

.

In the fourth century, the gladiatorial games were replaced by Christian matrimony; the amphitheater was replaced by the bedroom—the bourgeois theater.

.

Women's skirts are a parasol that shelters us from the cruel rays of life. (Women in trousers: our skulls are bare.)

.

Only a sense of honor can prevent the worst iniquities of natural egotism. Some people are naturally good and generous; but those who are not born that way have only one restraint, the product of upbringing and practice. If I do this, if I do not abstain from this, if I turn back, if I do not go, if I eat everything, *I dishonor myself in my own eyes* and shall be punished by Shame. Thus self-love, noble attachment to the ugly pronoun that designates us, remains the only salvation in the storm of the amoral I's vile hungers.

.

Monstrous, untarnished egotism always finds some adoring woman. Limited, controlled, cautious egotism, which strives to restrain itself, arouses intolerance, because it does not cover, it does not submerge, it does not engulf everything.

.

The obsession that one is being persecuted by an organ, by one's own bowels, nerves, vertebrae, joints, veins, skin, and weight, has become universal. The classic persecutors, Life and Time, are never mentioned.

•

There on the pier, stabbed by an ice pick, the Empress Elizabeth, symbol of the oldest European monarchy, which must die by a villainous hand. The contemptible Lucheni raved about making noise and killing someone in the public eye. But it was really the enduring vagabond melancholy of Elizabeth Wittelsbach that, in the mysterious dialogue of souls, summoned the madman to Geneva from Piedmont and anointed him as her assassin. For that matter, even the Italian government was a Lucheni. (Perhaps in its death wish, Vienna itself summoned him.)

•

The elderly take horrible revenge on the young for wrongs received at their hands, lighting thousands of nuclear fuses under their feet.

•

One of the most terrifying thoughts on human crowds, boundless and uncontainable, is that they are devouring mouths; one of the most discomforting is that they are intestines that do not shit. I have this philanthropic obsession . . . The urban, urbanized, enclosed, tarred, enshrouded crowds— Babelized in the brotopolis, deprived of any direct relationship with the earth, with the land, and with that which descends as seed and ferment from between the teeth of the ironic *Adamah*—are denied the ability to empty the intestine properly and regularly. The sitting position on the detestable hopper is the enemy of reasonable evacuation. Then there is the continuous goad of schedules and commitments, anxieties, neuroses, social inhibitions ("I couldn't, I was with them"), transfers, changes of environment, entertainment, loss of movement, work in closed spaces, and enormous greed. We coexist with robots whose waste bears no resemblance to our own (and hence offers no example, while the sight of a horse defecating stimulates evacuation). We eat dry, phony, un-slippery food, and are always on the go. The cities are im-mense stockyards of hardened, constipated bowels. It's enough to prompt sympathy for cities and their people . . .

The bladder is doing no better, but it is more readily obeyed, since it is easier to satisfy than the intestine. Some people forget all about their intestine. The great master is the ass, said Luther at the table. But the universal loss of desire for either God or master also takes the form of an absurd revolt against the Master Ass, who rewards proper treatment with days that are free for greater unhappiness and concentration. Tell me how many occasional sufferers of con-stipation (regular sufferers form a millennial knighthood), how many neo-constipants, can be counted in a modern cap-ital and you will have the most important X-ray of society.

The coprologist considers the fecal matter of urbanites to be of poor quality. Thus their fundamental treatment should be to free themselves of it as soon as it is formed. It seems we can animate this languishing function only by *worrying about it*. But straining to think about evacuation, focusing on the exoneration of the bowels—the only alternative to teas and suppositories—is harmful because it depletes nervous energy (better put: Psyche's exhausted fluid) from the activ-ities that free us from our enslavement to the bowels.

Thinking too much is exhausting, even if it makes the job go smoothly. The effort that goes into ten bowel movements could heal a pair of paralytics, communicate several dreams from Europe to America by telepathy, and levitate a person in the kitchen like St. Theresa. A strict mystic would call it thought taken away from God the Creator and given to an unsatisfying creature, making the intestine almost a coddled creature within a creature. And we are filled with regret, robbed of all other thoughts, when we imagine how much God has been stolen from us by this snake-like, voracious, obscure creature.

.

On the one hand, the constipated metropolises; on the other, the dysenteric concentration camp. These are the parallel creations of this century's lovely revolutions: the crowding that hardens the bowels, the crowding that dries them to death. A liberated survivor, man reenters the city, where the transition from dysentery to constipation strikes him as a miracle of healing balance.

.

The true, naked vice of Gluttony is not the passion for quantity, or for refined concoctions, or for the superfluous magnificence or the blood-alcohol-sugar levels of food. These are caricatures—elements out of a moral painting, the stomach's ancient exploits, recurrent vulgarities, laughable horrors, and Trimalchian literature. Gluttony is an almost abstract passion. Its object can be humble and meager. But the vice is heralded by the joyous foretaste, the mysterious and tacitly frenzied anticipation independent of hunger.

Over on the table, a boiled onion with a little oil and raisins, a green broccoli stem cooked without salt, a raw egg, brown rice with parsley, a plate of macaroni without sauce, a bowl of toasted barley, a heap of white beans, polenta . . . The *grimoires* of Haute Cuisine do not even name these things. Incestuous palates shun such foods, but the *gulosus* in me blazes for them, and its flames are ferocious, while I futilely say I am not an ascetic to those who think I am. I am a failed ascetic (and maybe an ascetic failure too). A true ascetic resists better than Hippolytus, even if a hot onion broth shows him its breasts and navel. At the smell of garlic, one of the most churlish delights, he flicks his finger. The diabolic perfection of a hen's egg, just removed from boiling water, whose spermatic white was considered tasteless by Job (a hagiographer can make mistakes) and whose yolk suggests the flames of Hades, remains alien to his motionless testicles.

O Shiva on Mount Meru! O Greek fathers of the desert! The strength to say no, to fast while hot potatoes and piping hot tea are set on a table with a white cloth! (A dark cloth diminishes one's craving. Heat stimulates gluttony; cold food is less enticing, while frozen food is disgusting.) The Castilian word for craving is *gana*, an open mouth in Gothic etymology, a lusting tube in Latin (*canne*). The desire of desires resides in the gullet; it is the sole thought of the old man who has ceased to be master of his gullet, a spasmodic thread of the Lust for Life attached to a tube.

The monster attacks no matter how little food is available, provided it is *pleasing* (I speak only of gluttony, not hunger). For me an apple is enough, provided it is a russet. The fragrance of an apple approaches the nose; Gluttony writhes like a woman in labor. In fifty hotel rooms between the first and fourth floors—and by the light of the reflection from outside or of the single lamp provided by the Management— one hundred abdominal gullets (maybe one hundred and two) rub one another to squeeze out something vague and dejected. But in the calm of one room, the glutton extracts from his bag a cup of yogurt smelling of honey and cuts a slice of bread with a knife. *Gana! Tanha!* The Epicurean's *little* pleasures? The enormity of small pleasures! Totality of pleasure in small pleasures! Fantastic pleroma of tentacles in small pleasures! Infinity, abyss, the perdition of small pleasures . . .

The Silence of the Body

.

Egoism is a huge monster of which we all partake, but unequally. Lucky is he who has received only half a fingernail, even if it is a talon. When will egoism reveal itself whole? Could it be embodied in a single human being? Perhaps Napoleon was Egoism incarnate, in a terrible but not criminal version. Criminal egoism is quite common; there are numerous criminals, and Hitler's egoism belongs to this type rather than to the terrible. Jesus? Now, there is a messianic egoism, a Christ-like egoism, a devouring fire.

The devouring, medullary fire of a profound soul is what spun the Napoleonic mystery. Women love great Egoists, but Napoleon was not loved by them, because his egoism so far exceeded the common measure. He was loved by his soldiers, those great absorbers of egoism and its excesses on the battlefields of old. For them, this cold man emanated warmth. "Cold? Near you, my Emperor, I immediately feel warmer!" a soldier told him at the Berezina. Egoism that warms is a human mystery. Amid the ice and the feet tormented by the freezing cold, the great sacrificer emanated warmth . . .

Women love the little monsters of egoism (children, lovers, fathers, every kind of imbecile), not incarnations of divine selfishness (except for Jesus). Catalogues of insanity consist solely of various degrees of egoism: an expert on egoism is already a psychiatrist. To my vexation, I think I belong to the vast crowd of average egoists. Sometimes I can shake the monster from my eyes (or heart or back). Other times I am easily overcome and guided. I coexist with its portion in me and am constantly negotiating and signing treaties with it. When I lose, reason comforts me.

.

The *Mahabharata* says that for a soldier it is a *sin* to die of an illness at home; it is not a sin to kill the enemy. In the world of ritual, these maxims are quite right. They are valid for the last of the despised professional soldiers, who fight here and there, for the men enlisted in the *Tercios*, *Légions*, and Marine Corps. But we have disobeyed all orders: mandatory conscription has created huge armies of soldiers who are not true *soldiers* because they were conscripted. For them, it is a sin not to die at home, and to die, instead, of a disease contracted in war. Since warfare is not their profession, draftees can legitimately refuse to kill. Everything possible is done to hide this truth from men drafted in wartime, but the truth is a serpent that often bites conscripted troops in the heels. They know they are not samurai or even foreign legionnaires. Without the system of illegal coercion adopted by every government to force resisters into combat, draftees would not have the opportunity to act or suffer like soldiers.

·

For a Buddhist monk, taking a bath more than twice a month is a sin. Whoever does not perform dirty work, sweating excessively and exposed to harmful dust, would do well to heed this rule: one bath every two weeks. In this civilization of neuropaths, there are those who, without getting dirty, take two or more baths a day. Blanche, in Tennessee Williams's *Streetcar*, takes a bath every fifteen minutes. Many women, terrorized by propaganda against Female Odors, take a daily bath. These are sins of *limpieza demasiada*, excessive cleanliness, as Theresa of Avila calls them, and the indifference of bath maniacs to the universal waste of water caused by their madness is amazing. Water will take its revenge.

·

Moses Mendelssohn says that authority can only humiliate; it cannot teach. In him authority is rebellion against God and the Scriptures.

·

I had boarded a plane that was definitely going to crash, while my mother had decided to let herself die in the water. She was sitting on a chair several meters under, her head lowered, hair untied, resigned. I suddenly shook off the heavy torpor that made me accept all this, reached her underwater, and said, Quick, let's go back up. I took her by the hand and we rose to the surface. The plane was no longer there.

·

Malachy, the Bishop of Armagh, died at the home of his biographer, St. Bernard, in Clairvaux. Bernard recounts the miraculous healings Malachy performed. One of the simplest: he sent three apples to a woman afflicted with unstoppable bleeding; the woman was cured. The apple is a fruit that can be mysteriously manipulated by magic powers. In the tales of the brothers Grimm, the apple takes on the face of death and induces a drowsiness that causes Snow White to be buried alive. Touched by Malachy, the apple becomes hemostatic, reanimating. The apple reawakens our conscience, introduces the vexing notion of Good and Evil, and behold, Good and Evil are in the house of man. In Latin, apple is *malum*. Beware of hands bearing apples.

·

It is stupid of us to abhor and to curse necrophagous animals. Do we know them well enough? Perhaps they know the beauty of cadavers better than we. Baudelaire, the *vulture sublime*, intuited this beauty, which the clairvoyant of Ephesus, strangely did not see. He recommends throwing corpses out like excrement. When poor Bovary lifted Emma's veil, he was horrified by the abdominal stain, although he was a

213

doctor. But for the desert beasts, it may be a splendid moon reflected in the water, surrounded by swans and water lilies.

·

"Gentlemen, come in. Here are the chambers where the torture sessions take place: the biggest rooms, the corridors, the so-called elastic room, and the narrow passageway that leads to freedom, often at the price of unbearable pain. They are not always used. Many people pass through here indifferently and even pleasantly, without being touched even once. But at times someone makes a signal: That one there. The chosen one is stopped, and his torture begins. The instruments with which the chambers are equipped are not always sufficient: others are brought in from outside, perfected by a millennial art. Now the visit has ended. The place you have just seen is called the Male Urological Apparatus."

·

If a person believes in the miraculous signs manifested in the life of Pius XII—a life that hardly conjures up grandeur, despite the great opportunities offered by the times—his opaque tiara will emit beams of light. On the night of February 19–20, 1939, Pius X appeared to him predicting he would be Pope. But seeing Pius X was no great vision. Another vision was more interesting: one of the secrets of Fatima that Soeur Lucia das Dores, the clairvoyant from the Cove of Iria, revealed to Pius was that he, Eugenio Pacelli, was the last descendant of the Bourbon kings. (But which descendant was he of the many who wandered around tragically declaring that they were the last?) On December 2, 1954, in a seriously ill state brought on by one of his recurrent hiccup attacks, he had another vision, of Jesus himself. He immediately said, *Iube me venire ad te*, order me to come to you, but Jesus did not want to.

The Silence of the Body

His room was furnished with German furniture bought during the time he was Papal Nunciate in Germany. It must have looked gloomy against the ivory white background of the walls. His radio stood in for Poe's Raven. An antiseptic white telephone was on the night table. Inside a large dressing room there was exercise equipment and a mechanical horse for simulated riding. In the papal apartments there are three safes, full of the hands of Christian castaways and celestial promissory notes. Why did you choose this place to show yourself, Christ? The most extraordinary vision, however, was in late October 1950, when the Pope was taking a walk through the gardens of Castelgandolfo and saw the sun writhe convulsively, as in a Van Gogh landscape, and take the shape of the cross, as at Fatima. His successors were duller: Pius XII was the last to feel and love Miracle.

·

To all outward appearances, Trotsky's assassin died from cancer in Havana, but in reality he is a devil of average rank who will definitely be assigned new missions on the earth one day. Without knowing this, Marie Craipeau, who met Jacques Mornard in Paris in the company of Sylvia Ageloff, portrays him as a perfect devil. The handsome Jacques's name was not, of course, either Jacques or Mornard, and perhaps not even Mercader, his official identity's last resort. He is a true storybook devil: handsome, charming, superficial, never short of money although he did not work, seducing weak spirits (like Sylvia) but making strong spirits grow tense with an undefinable suspicion. Something about him isn't quite right, and yet . . .

He moved easily from one continent to the next: in New York he was loaded with dollars and in Paris with francs. His designated victim knew him by the name of Jackson. He succeeded, as only a devil can, in penetrating walls thick with rifles and guarded by suspicious eyes. At the right moment, the enigmatic fool carried out his mission: he dealt the blow of the fatal pickax. He was immediately welcomed in a maternal prison, where he spent several calm, serene years. In 1960 a plane arrived expressly from Prague to pick him up: his Soviet masters, not knowing that the handsome Jacques had been born untouchable, thought they had to protect their exemplary killer from Trotskyite vendettas. He would live for another eighteen years, a retiree who could not sit on a park bench and tell his stories like any other old man in the sun. *Come, thick night* . . . The spirits of evil, the occult ministers of assassination will not let him idle among the Manes for long.

.

Everything that touches Parini is noble and delicate, even the malarial fevers from which he suffered. "Oh powerful bark, oh rare gift" ("Ode to Quinine"). "I venture to write with uncertain hand to your Excellency from bed, where I find myself newly indisposed by tertiary fever" (to Count Carlo di Firmian). Milan was besieged by swamps and irrigated fields (*The Salubrity of the Air*). Today malaria in the Milan area seems like a small calamity, a scourge that could fit into a short verse, Parini's decorous lament.

.

Two lines from Horace:

> *nec desint epulis rosae*
> *nec vivax apium nec breve lilium.*

> *At the banquet let the roses not be lacking*
> *or the long-lived parsley or the short-lived lily.*
>
> (*Odes* I, 36)

The Silence of the Body

Everything pagan and classic, ancient and distant, seems to dwell in these lines, like a billion shadows in a closet. But to gain access to them you must first overcome much repulsion, especially toward the waxen, the waxified, the cadaveric, the mummy, and the lifeless human form wandering through apparitions like William Blake's, toward the torpid morgue of darkened bodies, the House of Death redolent of what Manzoni so pregnantly called "the mortal air of paganism." A friend returns from Spain and even the kisses he gives and receives are scenes from a private realm of the dead, from a Horatian House of Death, a Sheol without the tears of grieving Semites. These two lines form a perfect image of Western paganism and classicism as a temple of Death. They evoke Horace's art, the most literal *conciso*.

I am attracted by journeys (short, with quick returns, because long sojourns immobilize me) into the spirals of Horatian melancholy, where the *Conciso* (the Cut, the Broken, the Contracted) is the pale master. They represent a sure salvation after a person has cried *Eli, Eli* in vain. You cannot stay there for long if you have residues of passion for the infinite. Horace is saddened at having to sever his ties to infinity, to uproot and extirpate the infinite, the uterus of Sorrow, like a Leriche of the Aeolian lyre, and at having given himself entirely to Meter like a suicide to the rope. After killing the infinite, he goes into mourning, comforted by its disappearance but joyless. Ah, in those two lines that speak of a dinner set for mute faces, the mouth of paganism seems to be telling its unimaginable Christian successors, "You can't understand me anyway," silencing even their curiosity.

Yet in the Christian schools, where more Horace used to be taught than prayer, there was always murmuring and shuffling about before proudly locked doors such as this. But, Christians, if you break down these doors you will scream with horror. Behind them you will see the bodies of Horace,

Maecenas, and many others—Thaliarchus, Aristius Fuscus —some dressed, some naked, covered with roses, parsley, and lilies in a pool of spilled wine. *Rosae* and *lilium* are symbols of the ephemeral, but *vivax*, the long life attributed to parsley, pains the heart even more. Nothing could be more *cinis et umbra*—ashes and shade—than this dead *vivax* sprouting up between the roses and the lilies. What is *vivax* in the House of Death? The Master of Death, the rosebush of Thanatos?

In the Psalms there is a falling and rising movement around the tombs; in the Gospels and Revelation the sepulchers are never closed, never final. The paganism embodied by Horace nobly rejects the Tomb in Motion, the open-close-reopening of a Hades that has lost its gravity. Monophageous among friends with poor appetites, who nourish the roses' death and the funereal music, Horace does not allow at his table a breath or a shriek from tombs that give way and howl, nor the gravel from eschatological earthquakes. His is a surgical art. This unchanging calm (*epulis, rosae, apium, lilium*) is instantly a scalpel someone is twisting in your chest to extract something with effort and with considerable resistance from the penetrated cavity: a sensitive organ, a bloody sponge besmirched on the floors of the passions, a place of hammered nails and thrown knives. Behold, the chest is emptied, cleansed, lightened, and delicately dead: a dried carcass amid the bandages and perfumes of paganism, a condition that can well be considered enviable, for it shelters a body from the saponifying flies of unhappiness and of the present.

Bringing the scalpel crowned with *vivax apium* to the incision point, Horace the surgeon becomes a maternal Arria: "*Paete, non dolet*—Paetus, it does not hurt." In fact, it does not hurt. It is post-Socratic Nirvana, an imperfect Nirvana a few meters above the desperate boiling of the world, the unequal brother of absolute Extinction. It can be extremely painful not to surgically amputate the infinite from yourself

The Silence of the Body

once you have been remodeled in the finite and welcomed into the post-Socratic guest rooms to escape from the wounds of the world.

Koheleth, the Sadducean *afikòros* (wise man), can be imagined as a Horace who opens the door to infinity in each of his hundred houses. Behold his inconsolability when unleashed Infinity throws itself through the opening on the defenseless Finite—the Lover whose master is extremely jealous—corrupting and violating it without respite.

To picture the immortality of the Word, Horace saw his own work as a sepulcher: *aere perennius*, more durable than bronze, but still a House of Death.* He challenges Time and the water that erodes everything, but he is eviscerated, embalmed, and swathed. "Nec desint epulis rosae" . . . is what one sees from the window of the *monumentum*, the convivial tomb, the sepulchral symposium of immortal Horaces saved from Persephone (*vitabit Libitinam*: he will escape death) by a word that turns them into pyramids. A Renaissance architect like Brunelleschi comes much closer to *monumentum* than any Augustan ruins. No Roman ruins are Horatian; the Italian Renaissance interprets him much better. Renaissance is reproduction of tombs, imitation of sepulchers. The *Exegi monumentum* should be read in San Lorenzo or before the Pazzi Chapel, buildings erected like Horatian verse, without a single Christian vein. Brunelleschi was also post-Socratic Nirvana, an inflexible nirvanic surgeon who attracts and slightly repels me, House of Death, renunciation with no compensation other than a long, placated gaze at one's own amputation. But this man from whom the infinite has been amputated still kicks desperately and tears the waxen roses from his head.

---

* *Exegi monumentum aere perennius*—I have erected a monument more durable than bronze (III, 30).

Place these two lions opposite each other, one alive, even if a little mangy, the other of stone but proud: Miguel Unamuno, the muscular Christian, and Horace, the muscular classic, who for some time now has often been my Jonah's gourd plant. I want to live forever, shouts the famished Salamancan of living immortality in his *Del sentimiento trágico de la vida*, and to live, me, this poor "me" that I am and I feel myself to be, here and now! He gets down on all fours not to roar but to howl, excruciatingly, against death, crying "Yo! Yo!" By comparison, the *Exegi monumentum* is a silence full of dignity, but its smugness shows as much joy and vitality as a fetus in a jar. This wondrous verse really erects the monument, but what does it build there? A mausoleum—where life is missing, not the roses. "Y es que en rigor la razón es enemiga de la vida . . . Todo lo vital es irracional y todo lo racional es antivital, porqué la razón es esencialmente escéptica" (And it is because, strictly speaking, reason is the enigma of life . . . Everything living is irrational and everything rational is against life, because reason is essentially skeptical).

Satiated by reason, the insane hunger for eternity ("un hambre loca de eternidad") can create only a monument more durable than bronze, in reality a tomb. But it is inevitable that, as you grow old, there is less *hambre loca de eternidad*. Even death without a monument seems acceptable, so long as the pain of life ends. I have lived within these formidable rhythms. I have always been accompanied by the wailing of Rachel in Jeremiah, by the howl of some famous Christian beggar (Luther: "In truth we are but beggars"), and by the black classical sun that shines like *Shamash* behind a veil of mourning. By nature I tend to favor the third companion and to take my anguished leave of Jerusalem, but I have not yet said farewell.

The Silence of the Body

> *. . . et vigilis lucernas*
> *perfer in lucem; procul omnis esto*
> *clamor et ira.*

> *. . . keep the lamps of vigilance lit until day;*
> *banish all sound and fury.*
>
> *(Odes* III, 8*)*

And the lamps that keep watch until morning are another of paganism's funeral pyres. The morning when the lamps are silenced is the shore of post-Socratic Nirvana, Extinction without the infinite. Only the absence of life excludes sound and fury. *Banish all . . .* It is Life that wishes to distance itself. *Clamor et ira,* it is the jail of the Infinite, frenetic frothing of impotence, head beating against the iron walls until either the head or the walls break, and sometimes it is not the head.

Anastasis, Anastasis, cries the greedy, mysterious night surrounding the Horatian house, where the lamps endlessly keep watch over the sad table of roses and dead Maecenas and where Damalis, a cow lusted after by languid gazes, protrudes her stony breasts. *Anastasis, Anastasis . . .* Who are they? Who cries this way? The heads of children, doused with a bucket of messianic water, a sign of the light? Good spirits, souls in Purgatory, bodiless spirits waiting, vampires, or Lucifer's angels? . . . *Anastasis:* a Greek, a very Greek word (if understood in all its ambiguity: destruction-resurrection, demolition-elevation), in this house where even the dead, the roses, and the lamps speak Greek. It is an unknown word, or better yet, a word of no account.

—Who is it?

—*Anastasis.*

The master of the house will send no one to open.

Postscript

If you medicate, meditate.
If you meditate, medicate.

I cannot understand the good fortune of what Roberto Calasso so generously described as my "fascinating scrapbook," but I must accept it, though mindful of the customary obscurity and willfulness of Fortuna's motives. For the reader the charms here are few, yet none of my books has been more successful—it has even set down on other languages! No amount of scheming on my part could have brought this about. What's even stranger, I myself hardly felt my little barques were fit for navigating unknown craters.

Of the various descriptions of this work, my personal favorite is "a satirical booklet." It came out in 1979 and still finds readers, some of whom write to me . . . And here I am, alive, meticulous, and rewriting. For the publication of a tenth-anniversary edition, I tried at the very least to revise and recolor the text and to offer both new and old readers little novelties, the results of self-criticism and of further meditation, stitched here and there into the settled fabric.

For years I have been fascinated by medicine, whose company I have kept in books and in my obsessive worries over health. Today (I have the distinct impression) it has come to defy all historiographic and speculative, not to mention ethical, supervision. Given the impossibility of forcing medicine back inside moral boundaries, thought, the assailant, strives to *understand* its terrifying object—the true Leviathan—by photographing from various angles the shadow cast upon the earth by this deadly comet. This comet is distinct from our other, everyday, every-hour Halley's comets, though sometimes they tangle and are confused in their fatal orbits around this silent globe.

I am appalled by the passiveness of bodies, of our unhappy lives, of our mortal bodies, under the scourge of Medicine's will. And I am dismayed by Medicine's insatiable omnipotence, its desire to do everything it decrees *for our own good*, making us wholly dependent in johnnies that look like they came from a concentration camp.

We have lost count of medicine's burglaries, violations of the flesh, demolitions, break-ins, barnstormings, kidnappings, black-mailings, consensual interceptions, rivers of black, white, and red blood, devastations, and cosmic robberies of both private and public money. Thought does not know in which category of evil to place it or how to digest so much pediatric blackmail, so much oncological, geriatric, obstetric, and cardiological blackmail, madly spread wherever there are doctors, health-care services, hospitals, laboratories, and clinics for chronic illness. Every bit of medical blackmail (which is sometimes attractively *affectionate* but always profoundly brutal) corresponds to a genuflection by the body's scapulas and mental vertebrae, the immediate surrender of the whole to a cease-fire order delivered to a part that is under assault, or supposedly about to be assaulted, by pain.

Molière's *Imaginary Invalid* is more distant than a star; all the old satires on doctors and medicine (until Jules Romain's inimitable *Knock*, which marks a turning point and looks to the future) pounded away at *human* defects, cynicism, ridiculousness, and superstition. But no satire can rail at medicine *like ours* (we are unprepared, we still know too little, we are only beginning to understand); it governs us, elusively, over almost the entire earth.

Postscript

Any university doctor is an armed and shielded giant, against whom the defenseless body-dwarf cannot do battle. Little does that doctor know that a little recalcitrance might be helpful, even beneficial, might have an ethical importance, a healing energy.

The depth of devastation wrought by medicine's retaliation cannot be weighed against the immensity of its concessions—relief from pain. Thought is tortured by the appalling uncertainty of medicine's moral pretexts and paralyzed by its triumphant results. If we even attempted to assess the damages, our heads would be left spinning.

IDOLATRY: Therein lies the only sin that gave goosebumps to the prophets of Israel and of Judah.

There is no need for a jailer: one need only use letterhead stationery and a telephone and behold the creation of interminable lines of worshippers in an unending pilgrimage, bringing before the idol their daily offerings of chilled urine and blood sucked from the veins, of feces and vaginal secretions to be translated into algebra. On the appointed day, at the appointed hour, they reappear, anxiously awaiting the response of the Sibyl, whose cryptic speech dispels or draws nearer each worshipper's moment of death. —I have to be hospitalized in a week . . . —and there I am, suddenly with a woman who is "to be hospitalized as soon as possible." Seven, eight, ten lives are caught in a whirlpool, all flowing together toward an entrance that is open night and day, where the guards stand around smoking.

Thought cannot help us transcend our wretchedness, since we need to know more than we can. It cannot help us assess the blind damage to humanity, to our human truth of struggle and death, and to our ability to wage spiritual warfare brought about by the permanent removal of childbirth from homes and from midwives and by the practice of forcing people, with fewer and fewer exceptions, to suffer and die *in hospitals* (lest they meet sudden, violent deaths). This death cannot even occur in beds meant for rest, but more and more frequently in *rooms* designed for therapeutic ma-

227

nipulations, where the patient is penetrated by machines and intimately disfigured by chemical treatments. Indeed, the Hospital has appropriated the alpha and the omega of birth and death. One cannot even deliver oneself to a (mechanically) ascertained death: the funeral must take place *inside the structure*.

I can only say that, since my day is also approaching (a thrilling adventure derided and even *excluded* by the possible!), my anguish is increased by the fear that I will be unable to die at home. Nevermore will the bell toll. Instead, the ambulance's siren splits the traffic, announcing each time: "It tolls for thee."

We cannot even assess the loss represented by the steady annihilation of the *house call*. It has been replaced by the telephone, which at the established times icily dispenses prescriptions for drugs or dictates a future appointment.

Triumphant medicine could not have left us more alone, more ailing from the *lack of a hand* tapping that spot on the armchair where it rested forcefully so many times. We are left admiring its ticker-tape parades from behind iron bars of despair.

The hand, for beings who have them (Martians do not: will we lose ours?), is a microcosm of the grace that preserves and cures with inscrutable finality. This is where all the cosmic therapeutic currents gather, between the first phalanx and the rasceta, and (among those unmarked by sadism or idiocy) compete to generate the hand's secret energy, which can be increased through medical use, as it is in dance and mime. A doctor who does not carry his own hand, gracefully, into the sickroom (Munch's doleful drawings) is a destroyer of the body and will battle it with his snarling silence of resigned mortality, of undeciphered living dead. Unfortunately, the absentminded specialist will know nothing of this and feel no remorse for his days of full schedules with no openings.

Goya and His Doctor, Arrieta (so far away, unfortunately—the Minneapolis Institute of Arts) is a poem of humanity that cannot be contemplated without tears, a grateful tribute to the good doctor who places his arms around his patient's shoulders, coaxing the recalcitrant old man to swallow a potion; it is an amazing tribute. But where has Arrieta gone? Today, in all of America, who could say they have encountered an Arrieta?

Goya painted this scene as an ex-voto; in fact, it is a post-Christian ex-voto in a world of enlightened *afrancesados* (Francophiles). The physician is transfigured into visible sainthood, into a Rescuer for whom you rush to open the doors. In the shadows they were preparing the obsequies, but here is Arrieta, and the seventy-three-year-old Goya will once more succeed in standing up . . . Arrieta is awaited, even today, but what arrives instead is the ambulance: you will be shattered . . . In that haze of blood, atom among atoms, oh for your hand, Arrieta!

We cannot imagine the Hubris committed in the medical field or treat it as a calculable quantity, because these acts are *éminences grises* that accumulate without incorporating in order to manufacture destiny. The Hubrises coagulate to form what hermeticism calls "rule by demons"; they are active violations that become forms of sublunar life and assume leadership positions . . .

For a moment let us focus our attention on one point. The suffering that we cause animals used for experiments forms a chain of Hubris (a term I understand exclusively to mean a transgression of the impending and unrevealed moral law) covering all the Hellenism of this and other worlds with an icy pallor. Despite all its Greek vocabularizing of itself, and the invasions of American acronyms, Medicine has not found a way to annex *Hubris*, its basic *illness*, its flaw of power overstepping the Limit.

When the earth spews forth its stories, once again we shall see all the eyes of the weak creatures who were sacrificed.

But I wonder to what extent humanity, incurably *healed* by Western medicine, is now trapped by the rats it exterminates with such ingenious nonchalance in its laboratories. I mention only rats—though they are not alone in suffering the experimental madness masquerading as icy reasoning—because rats are the majority, and on the lowest level, the cheapest commodity, the one that least disturbs the conscience. In most, why not say all, prescriptions, the hand that writes is inspired by a rat. The rat rules over the shelves of the Pharmacy, and its clever little nose pops out of the white coats sashaying down the corridors cheerfully greeting one another. The little rodent gnaws gnaws gnaws . . .

The Body never wanted relations with the rat, the *rattus*, the dweller of granaries, sewers, and tunnels, the defiler of cadavers in watery places, the phallic symbol, the soiler of kitchens, the incubus of wells and prisons. Medicine forced it into this marriage, which takes place via drops, pills, and cosmetics, parenterally and rectally. Medicine wished to set the Body between the Rat's paws in order to restore memory and movement to the joints, to lower arterial pressure, restore sleep, dispel anxiety, set the intestines back in motion, and disinfect wounds. The rat blocks the thyroid gland, administers cortisone, shrinks the prostate, prevents pregnancy, banishes polio, washes our hair, and tightens wrinkled skin.

The modest mind of this tiny gnawer of living and dead paper is what makes today's historic decisions, winning and distributing Nobel Prizes in Medicine, assuming responsibility for peace and war, archiving the famous data without which knowledge would grind to a halt, and providing for the irreparable, devastating scientific locking of the gates to the world. A rat's skull stares at us from a rotting doorway.

There is something more powerful than a pandemic and analogous: a circle that was established from rat to flea and that determined human history. The influence of the rat on human existence (via pharmacological tests) introduces psychic and intellectual modifications unknown to Yersin's plagues. Today the rat nibbles at us from the depths of its unnatural suffering, from its tiny lazarettos of certain, excruciating death. It is more inside our lives than when its ancestors jumped off the docks and followed the caravans. Is not such research on cancer already *cancer*? Is not such psychiatric research already *madness*?

Is there such a thing as an AIDS of the mind—hiding, escaping, and falling from spiritual immunity? There are huge arsenals full of remedies—but what remedy is there *for this*? You can plug such a leak with a drug that gets rid of eczema in two days but compensates for its efforts by boring a hole in the stomach, where it deposits its formula and, after a brief period of usage, lays the solid foundations for the inevitable carcinoma! All treatment for the ailing *spirit* is administered by *matter* that acts as matter, that cannot grasp that which is foreign to matter but can modify it by ineffably acting on the body.

A chilling thought: The only things keeping the city from collapsing are analgesics, liquid anxieties, psychopharmaceuticals, sleeping pills, and sedatives; it does not collapse because it is sustained by the consuming worm's nest of legal and illegal drug addicts. Are they the Fifty Righteous Men? Or is the city sustained' because hidden in its sewers are ten unimaginable Righteous Men, with the beard of Shem Tov and the eyes of lost Sophia?

The truth is that the city's resistance is an unending collapse: it falls apart and the law retreats. Drugs can keep it alive only provisionally and desperately. Maybe the city is already dead, like Beckett's visionary in *Endgame* or the earth in Jeremiah 4:23–26. I also wonder where all the anxiety we repress but cannot extinguish ends up. In a Mississippi of urine? What chains of psychic sewage hold together each of these megalopolises (each with a mayor!) speaking English, Italian, French, Urdu . . .

Medical triumph is human failure because we have not found a less unfair way to overcome pain and old age and death.

Such a broad power necessarily employs many scoundrels, dreadful scoundrels with degrees in hand. Absolute probity lives uncomfortably there, and succumbs. The relative probities can only slightly attenuate the tremendous destructive energy of such a nonstop show of force.

There is fear of the body: see it in Eros confessing, in crime enthralled by obsession, and in medicine that has tamed and now observes the body. (The expression "under medical surveillance" is meant to be reassuring, but imagine, for a moment, being always *surveyed*, internally, by instruments—the thought makes me shudder.)

The overwhelming fear of the body is one of those ancient, ancient fears, adopted and never relinquished by Christian women (the Patriarchs' *De virginitate*, the confessors' manuals, sinister coffins . . .). It could not be diminished by repeated stormings of the Bastille from the eighteenth century on, or even by the decrease in infections. This fear belongs to the metaphysical terrors from which only death can deliver us. (In dermatology, observations of merciless interest can be made on this.)

What an error to think this fear is absent from contemporary medical power, that enormous, cannibalistic whale; it seems to have been erased from medical practice, but the will to subjugate is the fruit of fear. The secularization of death expands the desert: sacred shelter from decay. We also observe the symptom of fear-of-the-body in the specialized atomization of power. Medical specialization allows the physician to look away from the totality of the body and to avoid the bravery needed to know the body all over. A cavity is enough—the mouth, the uterus—and may the rest leave us alone . . .

In a certain sense our persistent fear of the body (and even of the frightened and thus less frightening infirm body) partially salvages the body-symbol, its otherness, and its evil powers (which do exist, and how!). This fear betrays a fault, an impotence, an unconscious weakening of the subjugating instrument.

The body manifests its fundamental restiveness in the mind's longing to reappropriate its lost magic power over the elementary spirits of infection and over parts of nature. But it is infinitely easier and more comfortable to enroll in a school and graduate brilliantly, to inspect the inorganic and the living world scientifically, than to become a *sorcerer* by developing the faculties that have been left to rot in the mystery of the body. This sorcerer could heal—as well as assist, gently and bloodlessly, whoever wishes to die—through the traditional knowledge of the intact but neglected sensibilities, the qualities and substances, blowing Yang into the dark Yin territories of aching matter.

The hunger for magic is quite reasonable. The risk is that malign Destiny will steer this hunger toward the star of evil. But today there is much greater need for *good magic* than for *good medicine*.

The relationship that science has forged with living and nonliving matter, with the soul and with God, is that of the psycho killer with his victims. Whoever wishes to be saved must never stop suspecting this, although it makes every inevitable dealing with doctors and their cures more *agonizing*.

The relative but undeniable success of certain organ transplants (outrageous Hubris) has forced the underworld gods to withdraw completely. The rights of the living have been infringed by the introduction of laws that change, soften, and rattle the notion and legal definition of death. There must be enough death for the body to be taken and its vital organs removed, but not so much as to completely freeze the remaining pulse of life in the organs destined to emigrate, on long journeys, to a body freed of its own useless or ailing organs.

Medicine is thus about to take one more step toward becoming the absolute judge over life and death. Every government is adjusting its laws. As in the myth of the Minotaur, the idol commands and must be served immediately.

A few more years of this incredible fin de siècle, the most crucial of them all, and every aspect of manipulating living cells and bodies declared *usefully* dead will be legal. At the same time there will be a feverish shrinking of the ethical and conceptual boundaries on being dead. I wonder how we will be able to stop criminal organizations willing to serve the (growing) demand of the market by providing clinics buried deep in the woods with tender young bodies deliberately sacrificed—here and there, darkness on darkness, in the poor and defenseless world. To operate on the dead, the demonically possessed will make use of computerized accounting and of other doctors inured to massacres, like Petiot.

This could become a traffic that is almost tolerated, indeed— like today's drug traffic, over which evil has absolute rule—barely disturbed by modest legal persecutions. I could hardly imagine it if I did not know that such events already occur, behind a shifting gray curtain of blood . . . The *hour* will arrive when Modern Medicine will overcome death—the mortality at the essence of man's being. For sixty interminable minutes, over all the inhabited earth, in a compact darkness never before seen, there will be a tremendous silence. No one will rejoice: for one hour everyone will be *prisoners of life*, materially a-mortal but not (ever) *Dii immortales*, amid the criss-cross and cascade of American and pontifical voices. It will be the true, the supreme *heart of darkness*.

February 1990